THE OSTOMY BOOK

BARBARA DORR MULLEN

KERRY ANNE McGINN, R.N.

THE OSTOMY BOOK ❖ *Living Comfortably with Colostomies, Ileostomies, and Urostomies*

BULL PUBLISHING COMPANY   *Palo Alto*

iii

Illustrations: Susan Klug

© Copyright 1980
Barbara Dorr Mullen
Kerry Anne McGinn

Bull Publishing Co.
P.O. Box 208
Palo Alto, California 94302

ISBN 0-915950-41-3
Library of Congress
Catalog No. 80-66390

Dedicated, with affection,
to everyone who has an ostomy—and
to all those who care for them.

Contents

Dear Reader,

This book happened because Barbara, a free-lance writer, had a colostomy. And was curious. Why didn't anyone talk about ostomy surgery?

Barbara's daughter Kerry, an R.N. and an experienced writer, joined the project later.

For two reasons, we believe The Ostomy Book *is a rather special book.*

First, so far as we know, it's the first book for the general reader on ostomy surgery, a group of abdominal operations which save thousands of lives every year, yet remain wrapped in secrecy, taboos, and nonsense. It's time the windows were open.

Second, it's a book that's had such an enthusiastic group of helpers, lay and professional, that it's almost embarrassing to put only our names on the cover as authors.

After joining the United Ostomy Association, Barbara sent a plea for help to the central office. The results were beautiful and overwhelming. Ostomates from all over — Nova Scotia, New York, Chicago, Medicine Hat, Texas, California, the Oregon coast and elsewhere responded with letters, personal accounts, and newsletters. The message was clear — we need the book. One of our favorites came from Muriel Bastin in Monterey, California, who told us that she's well enough following her ostomy surgery to drive her pink Buick again and says she's just gotten her driver's license renewed — at age 94!

We are grateful to David Bull, our enthusiastic and supportive publisher; Susan Klug, our talented illustrator; and Gloria Fisher, our dedicated typist.

The following people carefully reviewed the manuscript and enriched it with their wisdom and information: Victor Alterescu, R.N., E.T. (Victor has recently changed his last name from "Alter"; when he made the statements quoted in the book, he was still Victor Alter.); Donald Binder, Executive Director of the United Ostomy Association; Gerry Cameron, R.N., E.T.; Catharine Flinn; Katherine F. Jeter, Ed.D., E.T.; James R. Kirkpatrick, M.D.; Edith Lenneberg, E.T.; Lotte Moise; Karen Moise, R.N.; Carol Norris, Ph.D.; Robert Reinker, M.D.; George Schreiber, M.D.; Valerie Stoller, R.N.; and Michael Wise, M.D.

We also thank the many persons whose stories appear in this book (and the Ostomy Quarterly *for permission to reprint several of them), and the many people who shared their experiences with us in letter and conversation. Without them, this book never would have come to be.*

And finally, we are grateful to Kerry's husband, Art, and their children — Michael, Kathleen, John, and Steven — for unbelievable patience with the book.

Fondly,

Barbara Dorr Mullen
Kerry Anne McGinn
April, 1980

CHAPTER 1 ❖ *I'm Going to Have a What?*

A human body is an ingenious assembly of portable plumbing.
Christopher Morley

As my friend Tom says, you never realize how many yellow cars there are—until you buy a yellow car.

Until July, 1976, I had no idea that hundreds of thousands of Americans had gained longer lives, thanks to a surgical change I'd barely heard of—an *ostomy.* Nor did I guess that I'd be one of the lucky ones who would receive such a bonus of time.

Nor that I would need it. . . .

Though the apple trees and primroses probably bloomed on schedule that spring, I'd been too busy focusing on black clouds and mud puddles to notice them. My work wasn't going well, my body seemed to have lost its bounce, and I'd been in a rut so long I felt bruised. If I could swing it, maybe a vacation—a week or two on Puget Sound—would help? What I needed was a change.

What I got was changes. Instead of two weeks moseying up the coast to the Sound, I got four weeks and two days in a pink hospital room with a distant view of Golden Gate Park. Instead of fresh salmon and wild blackberry pie, there were bland, hot cereal and jello on blue plastic trays.

Those changes were temporary. I also got a slight change in my plumbing—a *colostomy*—and that's permanent, but less trouble than I expected, and cause for rejoicing. No matter what I used to think!

It all started on a Wednesday in July, near the end of a long-postponed physical. That had gone well. The doctor, Michael Wise, and I were pleased at my rich blood, marvelous blood pressure, all kinds of good signs.

Until that undignified last lap. My body was bent like a tent on the examining table so Dr. Wise could look into my rectum through a special tube called a *sigmoidoscope*. He'd been talking to put me at ease. Then he stopped. After our banter, the silence was scary.

"There," he said, after a few moments. "Just relax a minute, Barb, while I get someone else to look at this." Someone else was a doctor who specialized in problems of the digestive tract. He agreed the small odd growth looked suspicious. They'd better do a biopsy; they snipped out a tiny sample of the suspicious tissue, so that it could be examined under a microscope to see what was causing the changes.

When my daughter Kerry and I returned Friday morning for the results, a cup of coffee (a welcome if ominous courtesy) was waiting for me. Dr. Wise didn't mince words. The sample tissue appeared to be maverick—a young cancer. "So—we want you to come back early Monday morning, ready to stay a week or two. We'll do a few more tests and then—probably—surgery."

"What kind of surgery?"

"A colostomy."

A colostomy! I didn't like the sound of that, though I wasn't really sure what it was. Besides, this whole business was absurd! My digestion had always been excellent. Other people got intestinal flu or worried about irregularity; I hadn't even taken a laxative since I was ten years old.

Yet, if I'm honest, it wasn't a total surprise. There'd been small omens, all that spring. In March, I'd made a note in a journal: "Some concern about bleeding from the bowel. Try to avoid *all* raw and rough foods and see if it goes away." Later in the month, I added a happy P.S. to myself: "Gone away. Probably just minor."

Even such brief interest in my bowels embarrassed me, I remember. I'd had the usual childhood indoctrination in things we don't talk about. Later, reading Freud had persuaded me that concern with elimination was a dangerous symptom of regression to a childish stage and not (as I know now) intelligent attention due the only body I've got. But, though I tried to ignore them, there were small continuing problems in April, May and June. Not much blood but some.

Of course I knew a change in bowel habits is one of the seven danger signals the American and Canadian Cancer Societies warn us about, but that couldn't mean me. I had enough trouble without worrying about that. . . .

"Any questions?" Dr. Wise brought me back to July.

"No." I had a million but couldn't find the words.

All that weekend, melodrama, numbness, and a small trace of common sense fought it out. I didn't know much about hospitals, and remember wondering silly things. Could I develop film there? Take my typewriter? I tried to stuff Saturday and Sunday so full of friends and chores I couldn't think about Monday, or touch my fears. Still, I wrote a few frightened farewell letters to old friends. "I'll be OK," I sniffled, "probably . . . although the doctor does suspect cancer. . . ."

When I checked into the hospital Monday I felt fine, though unreal—the stand-in for a documentary film, starring someone else. Further tests would show how wrong they were, and I'd go home. But more tests all said the same thing: rectal cancer, young but growing and dangerous.

I still didn't believe it.

Surgery would be the next Monday. Besides frequent visits from my daughter and her family, three other things cheered me during that week of waiting.

Recently, I'd finally read *All Creatures Great and Small*. Inspired by James Herriot's account, I found myself identifying with the animals he'd treated. As doctor after doctor examined me, remembering that book helped. I was less a person brought low by a vast dose of bubblegum-flavored castor oil than an ailing cow with the scours.

The day we'd gotten the diagnosis, Kerry (with some faint memory of an organization for people with this peculiar surgery) looked in the phone book under "Colostomy," called, and learned that the Golden Gate Chapter of the *United Ostomy Association* met that very night in San Francisco.

Though I didn't go with her, that meeting cheered us both. "They're an amazing group," she reported, "men and women of all ages, great fun, and most of them seemed to feel great." Kerry had won two prizes at the meeting—a new dish towel and a bottle of champagne. Good omens. Not so much winning as discovering that people who had ostomies were lively enough to think of things like prizes.

One of the women had convulsed them with a story from her trip to Hawaii.

"You mean people with *ostomies* travel that far?"

"You know they do. And anyway, that's not the point. This gal had always wanted to go to a nude beach, even before her surgery, but she'd never had the nerve. In Hawaii, she decided to risk it, wearing just a camera over her shoulder and a daisy-sprigged ostomy pouch on her belly. She'd worried about what people would say; the only comment was, "What a neat way to carry your film!'"

That silly happy story heartened us all week, and there was hope as well as information in the brochures Kerry had picked up at the UOA meeting. I read them until they were limp—stained with coffee, and probably a few tears.

Basically, I learned, there are three common types of abdominal ostomies. All are surgically constructed detours in which a channel of elimination is rerouted, so waste (feces or urine) is expelled through a small new exit, the *stoma*, in the abdominal wall.

In a colostomy—the commonest and the kind they said I would have—part of the colon is removed or disconnected; all or part of the rectum may be removed. The end of the remaining colon is brought to the surface through the skin of the abdomen, folded back like a turtleneck, and stitched in place. Cancer of the colon or rectum is our most common internal cancer and is the most frequent reason for a colostomy, but there are others. This surgery, the UOA brochure promised, saves lives or makes them longer than they would be without surgery. Now that I've met some people who've had their colostomies for twenty or thirty years, I believe it.

An *ileostomy* is sometimes performed for severe *ulcerative colitis* or other *inflammatory bowel disease*. In this case, the entire colon is removed or disconnected, and the end of the small intestine is used to construct the stoma. The result, like a miracle, is often an instant cure.

The third type of ostomy is a *urostomy* or *urinary diversion*. In this operation, the bladder is removed or bypassed and urine is redirected to an *appliance*, a leakproof, external pouch. This surgery can be done to extend life or cure disease. Sometimes it is performed to end months or years of embarrassing dribbling of urine.

Before surgery, I was less interested in all these anatomical details than in hearing about the lives people led after such surgery. Thanks to one sad true story I knew, I imagined I might be bedridden or at least housebound for a long time. This, I learned, was unlikely unless I was silly enough to choose to hide. People who'd had ostomies were skating, skiing, dancing, making love, and having babies. They swam, jogged, managed large corporations, preached, piloted airplanes, even rode Brahma bulls in rodeos!

And there were so many of them. Of *us*, I amended, somewhat tentatively. I'd thought such far-out, oddball surgery must be rare — I'd not heard much about it — but ostomies are common, commoner than surgery to remove a breast, for instance. Some estimate the annual total at more than 100,000 ostomy operations

I'm Going to Have a What? 5

in the United States and Canada alone, some temporary and some permanent, changes happening to people of all ages from newborn babies with birth defects to great grandparents with bowel obstructions.

Book learning is all very well, but right then I needed comfort and reassurance more than facts. My next piece of luck was remembering my friend Irv. Though I'd never asked for details, I'd heard whispers about some mysterious but life-saving re-arrangement of his intestines. An ostomy! Since Irv and a friend of his had stayed with me while they were on a bicycle trip that spring, I knew he was in grand health now, whatever they'd done to him.

Irv came to visit, as soon as he got my message.

"It's no big deal, Barb. Only another kind of challenge, and you like challenges."

"Some kinds. I like to pick them."

"Sometimes the unexpected ones are better."

"I hope you're right."

Prickly though I was, Irv's visit proved a comfort. So were other visitors, cards and calls and books and flowers. Reassuring, but still unreal. Why did *I* need get-well cards?

The surgeon, Robert Reinker, allowed plenty of time for us to talk the day before surgery, and was sympathetic as he showed me what they planned to do and where, drawing on my belly with a wide brown felt-tip pen.

"You'll put the darned thing low enough so I can still wear a bikini, won't you?"

"No promises but I'll try, Barb, and there are sexy one-piece bathing suits, you know."

Surgery was just like Marcus Welby, M.D. had taught me: three or four units of new blood, a tangle of tubes, overnight in the recovery room (more a precaution than an emergency). And enough drowse so it was still hard to believe they'd done anything at all—until I looked.

It took me several days to find the courage to do that. Under a bandage, a long and primitive-looking incision straggled up the middle of my abdomen. With those big black stitches, not even neat, I looked like a badly trussed turkey (though you usually use white string for that). I cried when I saw how they'd slashed through my once neat navel.

Slightly east of the incision, a small, clear plastic bag was adhered to my abdomen over the new opening, the stoma. Although this *thing* was both symbol and means for my new way of elimination, I found it harder to accept than the incision. It was so pink, almost watermelon color! Maybe, as it healed, it would fade? No, a stoma gets smaller with time but the color remains poster bright, the natural color of the intestine of which it's still a part.

Behind me, where my anus had been, I felt rather than saw another loosely basted incision, well buttressed with drainage pads. It hurt.

Looking at what they'd done finally made the changes almost real, and brought the first wave of sorrow out in the open. Sorrow and sometimes anger, splattering out in brief flurries over trifles. Why did this happen to me? I'd always eaten my spinach.

The tears embarrassed me, and so did the black moods, but I learned such grieving only *seems* irrational and childish — it's a necessary step in healing and accepting a loss. Until things healed a little, my body image was askew and my post-operative depression normal, even healthy.

In that drowsy post-surgical time, filled with assorted discomforts but little real pain, everyone pestered me to do a great many things I had little (though increasing) interest in doing. Walk up and down the long halls. Stretch. Breathe deeply. Finish your chicken broth. Smile. Swallow this. Swallow that. Turn over. Learn to take care of your stoma. I loved them all, or most of them, if only they'd leave me alone. . . .

But learning to manage my stoma couldn't be postponed forever. With any ostomy, we lose the muscular control we've depended on ever since we were first toilet trained. Regulating the bowels in one way or another is essential — physically, psychologically, and socially.

Though I'd read about the choices colostomates have, I balked at trying them. Dr. Reinker said he'd have an *ET* come to see me. From my cram reading I knew an ET is an *enterostomal therapist*, a professional who is expert in helping people learn to cope with all kinds of ostomies, assisting with both technical know-how and the psychological adjustment to being different from what we used to be. But why did I need an expert to teach me how to go to the bathroom?

Jean Alvers, ET, came that evening after dinner. The day had been one long sniffle, and I was stretched out, awash with melancholy, when she bounced in, smiling so warmly I thought she was ten feet tall! (Weeks later, I realized she's shorter than I am.) Jean has an ostomy, too; later I learned that she was one of the pioneers who'd helped develop the profession of enterostomal therapy, more than twenty years before. Now, there are more than 1,000 certified ETs in the United States and Canada. Real training centers have replaced early ingenuity.

With the help of Jean's spunk and know-how, I began to see an ostomy was not without hope, and even humor. And to believe problems could be solved, one at a time. The next morning when a nurse announced she was going to do such and such, I shook my head. "I'm going to do it; you may watch if you wish."

With help from what seemed like hundreds of people, I'd begun to reclaim my own body *and* my own autonomy. I'd stopped being the colostomy in the corner bed. I began again to be Barbara who had had a colostomy—along with measles, chicken pox, flea bites, sunburn, diphtheria, whooping cough, hepatitis, and assorted other maladies from which I'd also recovered. Strong though fuzzy convictions about my responsibility for my own body revived as I asked more questions, and balked some, knowing I had to be a working member of my treatment team.

I began walking farther each day, not because Dr. Reinker or a nurse said I must, but because I said so. The weekend before I was discharged, I dressed, picked up my two-hour pass, and went for a long walk, halfway round the lake in a nearby park. On my way, I stopped to marvel at every dandelion, every wind-bent tree, every ugly mutt chasing gulls. Part of getting well seemed to be rediscovering how wonderful life was, in spite of everything. Or because! The changes I'd had—and the risks taken—brought life into new focus. I began to sense what people meant when they said surgery could be a time of growth as well as pain, pain that was becoming harder and harder to remember, or even imagine.

Leaving the hospital was a bigger wrench than I'd expected, in spite of 5 a.m. blood pressure readings and other nuisances, and there were shaky patches in the weeks and months ahead. Unscheduled naps. Shaky legs. Storms of tears, blowing up out of nowhere. I didn't enjoy my first swim, or my second — but the third was great.

As for the *thing* part, soon I forgot all about it for hours at a time. Once in a while, I still look at it with surprise and even rare dismay, but it's far less trouble than I imagined and a small price to pay for life.

Though I'd worried some, friends surprised me. A few seemed embarrassed; most were supportive. Some asked about my revised plumbing with cheerful vulgarity. I found such plain speaking more helpful than shy whispers.

Judy asked so many questions as we soaked up sun on her deck one balmy afternoon, I finally asked if she wanted to see it.

"Yes," she said, dubious but determined.

When she'd looked, she seemed disappointed. "Is that all?"

Yup, that's it. The mark is a small one and, for most of us, the inconvenience is minor. That's just one of the things I've learned talking to many new friends, a number of whom just happen to be *ostomates* as well as horse breeders, joggers, writers of historical romances, commercial artists, teachers, water skiiers, undertakers, backpackers, and much else.

When I was ready, I took a trip, only instead of heading north to Puget Sound as I'd planned before surgery, I went south to San

Diego where United Ostomy Association's annual conference was being held that year. Almost 1500 of us from all over the United States and Canada, and from farther away — Sweden, England, Germany, India and Japan—gathered to compare notes and learn. And to rejoice because of the good things that had happened to us, thanks to slight changes in our plumbing.

Unhappily, not all ostomy surgeries have such satisfactory endings. More would, *if* they were done sooner. To insure that, we'll have to become more willing to listen when our bodies try to tell us something, instead of turning a deaf ear, as I tried to do.

And we'll have to get better at plain speaking. Openness about ostomies is still a critical problem. Celebrities and the media have been willing to talk about a *mastectomy* (removal of a breast), a *vasectomy* or almost anything else, but are not so ready to talk about an ostomy. The media features vampires, sixty-seven varieties of sexual pleasures and problems, all kinds of venereal diseases—you name it. Everything but ostomies.

It's silly, if you think about it. The upper end of the digestive tract is loaded with status, prestige—and profit. The success of gourmet restaurants, cookbook writers, fast and slow food chains, makers of lipstick and toothpaste attest to that.

The lower end is also loaded with profit—laxatives, diarrhea remedies, hemorrhoid remedies, toilet bowl cleaners, cutesy toilet roll covers, all are sold in our living rooms, via the euphemisms of TV. But, the minute food leaves the mouth and begins its many yards, life-building journey through the digestive canal, it's reclassified as hush-hush, the butt of third-grade jokes and four-letter words, no longer a subject for honest, open conversation.

I write about what happened to me because I believe secrecy about ostomy surgery can be as malignant as cancer; lives are lost in that kind of dark. Too many ostomates, shocked by the sudden changes in their bodies, don't know how much help is available. Unless they're lucky, as long as press, radio, and TV are largely silent, how can they find out there are trained professionals *and* trained volunteers, ready to help? Or clinics where problems can be solved? Easy-to-use appliances to contain body wastes, and conferences to lift their spirits?

Some don't learn soon enough that an ostomy is a chance worth taking. Victims of whispers, they postpone or refuse surgery which could have been life-saving, because of their own fears or (worse) those of their doctors, families, friends.

As Irv told me, that night in the hospital, an ostomy is only another kind of challenge. There aren't many limits on what we ostomates do, where we go, or the kind of fun we choose, unless we impose them ourselves.

I'm grateful for all my luck—early diagnosis, skilled surgery, good aftercare, and bushels of encouragement.

And delighted to report that this was a great spring for apple blossoms and primroses. They bloomed their heads off and, this time, I was watching.

CHAPTER 2 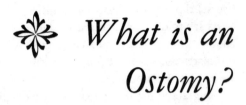 *What is an Ostomy?*

They say there's a well-preserved Egyptian mummy with what looks like an abdominal ostomy. Unfortunately, the physician left no record of why, or how, nor any clue about how it was managed.

An *ostomy* is a man-made opening into the body. An *abdominal ostomy* (the kind we're interested in) is the passageway a surgeon constructs through the abdominal wall as an exit for body waste—feces or urine. Such a change becomes necessary when the normal channel of elimination can not be used because of illness, accident or birth defect. A new outlet must be developed.

Ostomy refers to the total change the surgeon makes. *Ostomate* is one common term for a person who undergoes this change in personal plumbing. The new opening one can see on the abdomen is called a *stoma*.

There are three general categories of ostomies. A *colostomy* is the rerouting (permanent or temporary) of the colon (large intestine). *Ileostomy* describes such a detour in the ileum (the last section of the small intestine). *Urostomy* is a general term covering a number of different surgical procedures to redirect urine to the outside of the body when the bladder (or occasionally another part of the urinary tract) must be bypassed or removed, or when nerves do not control the discharge of urine.

More than a million and a half North Americans, ranging from infants to great grandparents, know what an ostomy really means —because they have one. Among them may be:

JOE, a newly retired engineer. During a check-up before a world cruise, he's shocked when his doctor discovers rectal cancer and schedules the surgery which will result in a colostomy. He's never heard of such a thing. It doesn't soothe Joe when his doctor points out that cancer involving the colon and/or rectum ties with lung cancer as the commonest cancer inside the body. (Well over 100,000 cases are discovered each year; it's usually a slow-growing cancer, though, and two-thirds of the deaths could be prevented with early diagnosis and treatment). What about Joe's cruise?

SUSAN, a beautiful and energetic toddler. The doctor explains that Susan's urine is not moving out of the body as it should, but is backing up to injure her kidneys. Other means to solve the problem haven't worked, so now Susan's doctor recommends a urinary diversion or urostomy. Susan's parents are horrified. Will Susan ever be able to lead a normal life? What will other children say?

MARCIE, a freshman in college. She's so miserable with severe bowel disease that her once-active social and academic life is now a memory, growing fainter each day. Even so, when her doctor says an ileostomy is necessary, Marcie weeps. Will anyone ever love her if she has such an odd change in her anatomy?

GEORGE, a young race-car driver. His colostomy is temporary, to give his large intestine a chance to heal after crash injuries, but that doesn't cheer him much. "How come I get such an oddball thing?" he snarls at the doctor, the nurse, and the hospital ceiling. "Bet I'm the only one . . ."

What is an Ostomy? 13

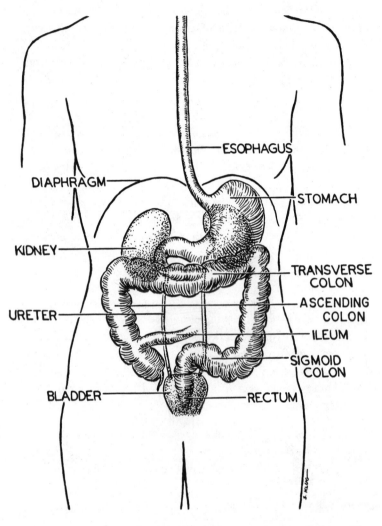

ESOPHAGUS

DIAPHRAGM

STOMACH

KIDNEY

TRANSVERSE
COLON

ASCENDING
COLON

URETER

ILEUM

SIGMOID
COLON

BLADDER

RECTUM

DIGESTIVE AND URINARY TRACTS. To make the relationships clearer, the artist has left out most of the small intestine, which twists and winds for 20 feet or more around the abdomen from the end of the stomach until the ileum, the last section of the small intestine, joins the large intestine (colon).

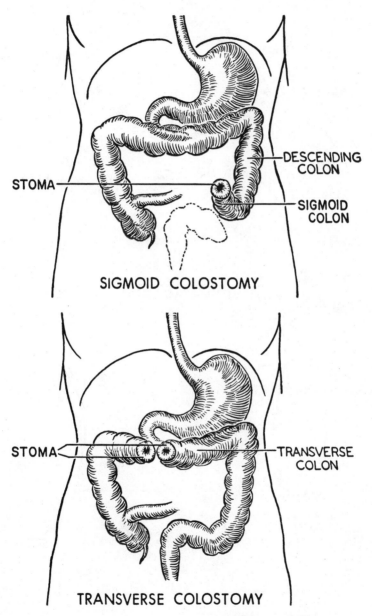

STOMA

DESCENDING COLON

SIGMOID COLON

SIGMOID COLOSTOMY

STOMA

TRANSVERSE COLON

TRANSVERSE COLOSTOMY

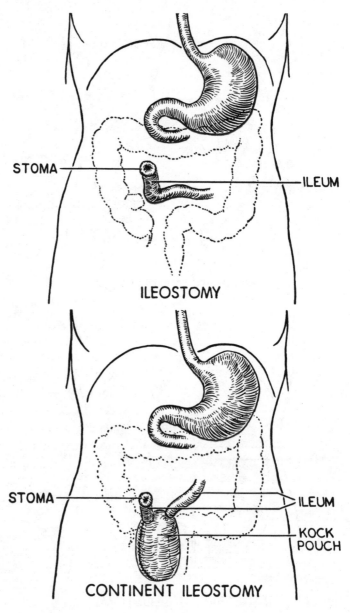

STOMA — ILEUM

ILEOSTOMY

STOMA — ILEUM

KOCK POUCH

CONTINENT ILEOSTOMY

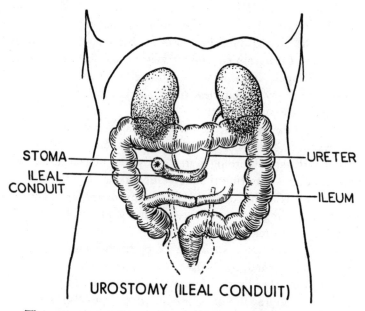

STOMA—
ILEAL—
CONDUIT

URETER—

ILEUM—

UROSTOMY (ILEAL CONDUIT)

The most common ostomies—colostomies and ileostomies—involve the digestive tract and depend for their success on its amazing ability to adapt to change.

Everything we eat, from apple pie and steak to pizza, yams, and zucchini, must be broken down into tiny particles and changed to simpler chemical substances which can be absorbed into the blood stream. The resulting nutrients make their way to cells throughout the body, thus providing constant fuel and materials for energy, growth, and rebuilding. This complex process of digestion takes place in the long (26 feet or longer in an adult) twisting internal canal known as the digestive tract, alimentary canal, or gut.

Digestion starts in the mouth, where food is chewed and enzymes in the saliva begin the process. From there, food goes via the esophagus to the stomach where churning action, different enzymes, and weak acid continue mechanical and chemical changes.

Becoming more liquid at each stage, the food proceeds into the small intestine, where substances from the liver and the pancreas further the process, breaking down even the most exotic foods into simple sugars, amino acids, and fatty acids. To be used by the body, the digested food must pass through the walls of the small intestine by way of countless tiny fingerlike projections (villi) which line the small intestine.

By the time food reaches the colon (large intestine or large bowel), most of the nourishment has been absorbed. Here the major tasks are absorbing water and some mineral salts, and transporting and storing the indigestible remains of the food in the lower part of the colon and the rectum. At the far end of the versatile winding digestive tract, the anus is a ring-like *sphincter* which opens to release feces.

The digestive tract is surrounded by smooth muscles which contract and expand, thus helping food move from one end of the tract to the other by the rhythmic waves known as *peristalsis*. These waves are almost constant; there are also stronger contractions, known as mass reflexes, which occur at the time of bowel movements.

Usually, the whole process of digestion is so automatic and so efficient that we forget its marvelous complexity (the liver alone has over 300 functions). As Thomas Fuller said, "Eaten bread is forgotten."

Occasionally, there is a massive breakdown in the system. The intestine may be blocked, completely or partially, by cancer, injury, or birth defect. Or food may rush through the digestive tract so quickly that there is little chance for nutrients to be absorbed; in severe inflammatory bowel disease, the person may be starving. In all these cases, an ostomy may become necessary.

The body adjusts quite nicely to a shortened digestive tract. If the ostomy occurs near the end of the digestive tract, as in most colostomies, the person has lost only a storage area, and a sphincter to release feces. If the ostomy is farther up in the digestive tract, as it is in a few colostomies and in ileostomies, the ostomate has also lost part of the ability to absorb water and mineral salts; thus the discharge tends to be less formed. But the remaining intestine eventually takes over some of this water-absorbing function, and the kidneys, the major regulators of water and mineral salts for all people, with or without ostomies, handle the rest of the adjustment.

Colostomies account for 65 to 75% of all abdominal ostomies. Since colo-rectal cancer, the most common cause for a colostomy, usually occurs in people over 50, and since it causes little or no distress in its early stages, most colostomates are over 50, and are surprised and shocked by what's being done. There's been no warning, or only such subtle hints as a change in bowel pattern, excessive gas, or a trace of blood in the stool.

In contrast, people who have ileostomies (which account for perhaps 10 to 15% of all ostomies) tend to be teenagers or young adults, and they've often had plenty of warning. Most have had a long or unusually severe bout with a fiery dragon of a bowel. Inflammatory bowel disease has laid them low with severe diarrhea (often bloody), cramps, and weight loss. In many of these cases, an ileostomy represents an instant cure. The colon has been a battle field; without it, peace is probable.

The final 10% of ostomies are urinary diversions, urostomies of one kind or another. After the kidneys have filtered wastes out of the blood, they flush excess fluid and wastes as urine through narrow tubes to an expandable storage area (the bladder) and then out of the body. At least some kidney function is essential for life, but any other part of the urinary tract can be removed or bypassed. Because reasons for urostomies vary from birth defects to cancer of the bladder, the age range here is wide, and many different surgical techniques are used.

In any abdominal ostomy, the damaged, diseased, or useless section of intestine or urinary tract is removed (or disconnected). To provide for the essential elimination of feces or urine, a new exit must be made.

In a colostomy or a standard ileostomy, the surgeon brings the end of the remaining intestine through the muscle, fat, and skin of the abdominal wall, forming a tunnel which folds back on itself like a turtleneck, and stitches it in place.

One variation on the ileostomy is the *continent ileostomy,* or Kock pouch, in which part of the small intestine is fashioned into a reservoir which is then attached to the inside of the abdominal wall. A slender tube, also made from the small intestine, leads from the reservoir out through the abdominal wall to become a stoma.

To construct an *ileal conduit,* the commonest kind of urostomy, the surgeon cuts a short section of small intestine away from the rest of the intestine, closes it at one end, and connects to it the narrow tubes leading from the kidneys; the open end of the disconnected segment of intestine is then brought through the abdominal wall as a conduit, or passageway, for urine to the outside of the body.

The stoma which results from any of these ostomies could be described as a soft valve. It stretches to permit waste to be expelled. During inactive periods, the tissue pulls together, rather like puckered lips (stoma, in fact, means "mouth"). Although it expands and contracts, the stoma does not have the firm muscle control of the anal or urinary sphincter; voluntary control of bowel movements or urination must be replaced by something else.

For many ostomates, an appliance is that "something else." An appliance is a man-made pouch, usually of thin flexible plastic or rubber, which is adhered to the skin over the stoma to hold feces or urine until a convenient time for disposal. An alternative chosen by many colostomates is *irrigation,* a kind of enema through the stoma, which permits them to empty the bowel at their convenience. They wear only a soft pad or a very small appliance over the stoma.

Since people with a continent ileostomy still have an internal storage area, they need no appliance; instead, they insert a plastic tube into the reservoir at regular intervals to drain feces.

****

Even though the view through a temporary post-op pouch may be a bit foggy, that first look at a new stoma in full, living color can be a real shocker.

In a note from Phoenix, Hazel Weathers wrote: "I wish someone had told me the stoma would be red. Red is the color usually associated with a sore or something unhealed. Although I did not have a great deal of trauma about the colostomy (I know you can't compromise with cancer), the first time I saw this stoma, I thought, 'My God, what did they do to me?' But it is now as much a part of me as my nose, ears or right hand."

Although the stoma usually shrinks slightly in diameter as post-operative swelling goes away and normal diet and exercise resume, the red color remains. This is logical, since this new exit is still a part of the intestine, lined with essentially the same kind of soft velvety mucous membrane as the mouth.

Unlike an incision, a stoma requires little healing. The stitches used are often the kind that don't need to be removed. A urostomy stoma starts to expel urine immediately, even before the new urostomate has left the operating room; the other types of stomas start discharging feces in a few days.

Stomas come in many shapes and sizes, depending on the kind of ostomy—and the person who owns it. Some are smaller than a dime in diameter; others are several inches or more across.

Shape varies as much as size. Some are round, some oval, and others are a bit irregular in shape. Most colostomies have the stoma raised slightly above the abdominal wall, perhaps ¼ to ½ an inch. Where drainage is more constant, as is the case with urostomies and ileostomies, the stoma is usually longer. From ¾ to one inch is said to be the ideal length. This length helps discharge waste directly into an appliance, instead of letting it pool on the skin.

At first, it's a temptation to feel over-protective about one's stoma, feeling it's so fragile it might be damaged by a draft of wind in the shower. While reasonable protection is essential, the stoma is surprisingly tough. It's not harmed by water, during sexual contact, or even by gentle bumps against furniture. It does bleed easily, even from as little cause as an overzealous swipe with a wash cloth, because many tiny blood vessels are very close to the surface of the stoma. An appliance or a soft pad will protect it from the friction of clothes.

Some stomas are constructed in the best possible location; others are not. Ideally, the ET or the surgeon (singly or together) spends time with the ostomate-to-be before surgery, watching how the shape of the abdomen changes when the person is sitting, standing, or walking—where the waistline is, where valleys and bulges occur. Then the probable site is marked.

If possible, the stoma is centered on a smooth and relatively flat plane, away from old scars or bones that protrude. Not all abdomens are ideal, however. Sometimes, because of fat or scars, there isn't any really good location for the stoma. And even with advance planning, the surgeon may change the site because of conditions discovered during the operation.

Within a few months after surgery, the stoma should settle down to a fairly consistent size, shape, and color. The shape may vary a little with change of position or activity, even coughing. Weight loss or gain (pregnancy, for example) may alter the contour of the stoma. But, different as stomas are from person to person, an individual stoma should look about the same from day to day, year to year. If the color or the shape changes much without an obvious reason (a too-tight appliance, for instance), it's time to check with a professional.

All intestinal stomas secrete some mucus, a thick liquid which helps lubricate and protect the intestine. As surplus mucus is discharged, it serves as a natural cleaning agent for the stoma. In addition, the skin around the stoma thrives on showers and baths, free of an appliance. However, scrubbing is not necessary and may hurt a stoma. A gentle sponge bath is another alternative.

Ostomates vary in their wish or need to nickname the new exit. In some families, the doings of Charlie, Rosebud, or Oscar are a shared joke. Margot Julian, RN, ET, has some questions about the practice. She feels nicknames depersonalize the fact and may interfere with accepting the change. "Does one name one's foot?" she asks.

On the other hand, few feet develop such distinct personalities as stomas do. In addition to their regular functions, they sometimes whimper softly, or sigh with unexplained contentment.

Especially at first, stomas may star in dreams or fantasies. This too, is "normal." It may help one work out feelings that cannot always be shared.

This takes awhile. Margot continues: "It seems like something that's been stuck on you, but it's been a part of you all your life. This is just the first time you've ever been able to see it. Sometimes it takes a while to think of it as part of yourself."

In the 18th and the 19th centuries, ostomies carried very high risks. With no anesthetics or antibiotics, patients clenched their fists and recited the 23rd Psalm. Mortality was high. With new techniques, surgical and postoperative risks are greatly reduced, especially when surgery is done promptly.

Although grouped under common headings, no two ostomies (and no two stomas) are exactly alike — each is a very personal thing. There are some new habits to learn but that's a small enough price to pay for an improved or extended life.

CHAPTER 3

❋ *It's Your Body*

NOTES ON JOINING THE TREATMENT TEAM

Sometimes good things happen in odd ways. About 6:30 that second morning in the hospital, I got mad — angry enough to weep and holler and, somewhat erroneously, call the surgeon a male chauvinist pig. . . .

The trouble started because I didn't feel I'd been accurately informed about a certain diagnostic procedure. Although I wasn't exactly proud of weeping like a frustrated four-year-old, that early morning storm served a purpose. After it, my surgeon and his colleagues took greater care explaining just what was happening, and why. Bit by bit, I became a functioning member of my treatment team.

Despite an early tonsillectomy and having a baby, my knowledge of hospital procedures was scanty. However, I knew I had some responsibility for my own body. Yet — unless I knew what was going on — how could I accept any part of that responsibility? What were they doing, and why? What would the results be? What were the risks? The discomforts? Did I have any choices?

Fortunately, my sense of personal responsibility coincided with great changes sweeping the health care fields. For many reasons, old ideas about physicians and surgeons as remote and omnipotent beings whose slightest word is Holy Writ, and compliant, quavering patients with a vocabulary limited to "Yes, doctor. . . ." are being replaced by something much more like a partnership—to everyone's benefit.

Doctors, nurses, and patients are becoming more aware of patients' rights *and* responsibilities, and of the very real contribution each of us can make to our own healing. In part, this change results from a better-informed lay public and greater emphasis on patient education, in part from the impetus of the holistic health movement, and in part from the medical profession's growing awareness of malpractice hazards. These forces, along with some intangibles, have resulted in the age of informed consent (in some states, there is legal backing for this).

For a long time we've known that patient attitudes may have a crucial effect on the healing process. That brave young fellow in room 517 on Ward E who makes it despite the odds is almost a cliché of fiction (and TV dramas); actually, such stories have a firm basis in fact and appear more and more often in the medical literature. Not all cures can be traced to Wonder Drug X. The individual who wants to live has the best chance of doing just that and, even with the best care, the patient's contribution—positive or negative—can make a difference.

Flora, one of our friends, happens to have two ostomies, a urostomy and a colostomy, plus other complications. She's an active and glowing woman; she is also a trained UOA visitor, a volunteer with an ostomy who visits people shortly before or after their ostomy surgery, passing along the news that a good life is possible after an ostomy. A few months ago, she was called to visit a woman scheduled to have ostomy surgery the following week. Unfortunately, despite Flora's obvious well-being and happiness, the patient muttered, "I'd rather die than have that happen to me." She got her wish—she died on the operating table.

While there may have been other factors involved, we believe that her unwillingness to take a chance on the proposed change, her reluctance even to try life with an ostomy, may have had quite a bit to do with her premature death.

Major surgery is scarcely a do-it-yourself project, and ostomies are major surgery. I didn't have the knowledge to order the necessary tests, nor the expertise to interpret them, but I could listen. I couldn't scrub for surgery or do a physical examination, but I could say "yes," "no," "maybe," "why is this test necessary?" —or even "I'd like a second opinion."

The patient's rights to information and a certain level of care have been spelled out in a Patient's Bill of Rights, presented by the American Hospital Association and reprinted after this chapter. Copies of these rights are given to patients at some hospitals upon admission.

The brave words in the Patient's Bill of Rights form a good working beginning for a team approach. They are honored more by some hospitals and physicians than by others. Some still prefer the old way and far too many patients throw away their right to know what's happening, letting the medical profession carry all the responsibility, no matter what their bodies whisper. Sometimes, though, they whimper to themselves, a roommate, a visiting spouse or friend, "I don't know what's going on. No one tells me anything." But they don't ask—and that's plum crazy.

Along with the right to ask questions goes the right to receive clear answers in words the patient knows and understands. From asking what's happening and what it means, or listening when an explanation is offered, it's not such a long step to asking sometimes, "What can I do to help?" or even, "I wonder if we could try. . . ." Participating doesn't mean constant demanding or gluing one's finger to the call bell, but it does mean awareness and some positive effort.

For the prospective ostomate, the treatment team seems almost as big as the production crew for a movie. (How, I wondered, could all these strangers know so much — and seem to care so much—about *my* gut?)

The team includes not only the ostomate-to-be (hopefully),

but also the surgeon, his assistants and other physicians (in a teaching hospital, where doctors spend one or more years after medical school learning under the supervision of more experienced doctors, this can mean quite a number of people). It also includes nurses. Around the clock, they're still the bulwark of treatment, including sophisticated specialists who limit their services to the operating room or recovery room, as well as timid student nurses, as excited and apprehensive as you are about seeing their first ostomy.

There are also respiratory therapists, x-ray and lab technicians, anesthetists, dietitians, social workers, sometimes physical therapists, ward clerks, maintenance people and volunteers in crisp starched pinafores. Of great importance to many patients are the hospital chaplains.

Family and friends are ex officio members of the treatment team; they can help or hinder—depending in part on their level of information, in part on your rapport. However well you know each other, people are full of surprises in unexpected situations. Sometimes friends or family have unpredictable reactions, or repeat old wives' tales best forgotten. But, along with fruit, a paperback mystery and a bunch of daisies, they also bring hope.

Other patients (and their visitors) are often helpful, counteracting your anxieties with a rousing tale of what a great life their Aunt Alice has had since she had her ostomy, fifteen years ago! While hospital friendships are sometimes as brief as shipboard romances, the support and companionship of others who are not strangers to early morning temperatures and bedpans can be very heartening.

And, high on the list of team members, are trained visitors from the United Ostomy Association. It really helps to talk to a man, woman or child who owns an ostomy, and enjoys living.

Important, too, are both the moral support and technical know-how of an enterostomal therapist (ET), a specialist in how to deal with this slight change in one's plumbing. Of both UOA visitors and ET's, we'll have much to say later.

For any ostomy, the forecast varies—from excellent to poor (or, as they say, 'guarded'). Not all of the results are controllable. If, for instance, colo-rectal cancer has been discovered too late, surgery will probably result in increased comfort but not necessarily in longevity. As taboos fade, and early diagnosis becomes more the rule, earlier surgery will bring with it a brighter picture.

In any case, no matter how many big-name specialists join your treatment team, without you they're not going to make medical history. With you on the team, who knows?

PATIENT'S BILL OF RIGHTS

1. The patient has the right to considerate and respectful care.

2. *The patient has the right to obtain from his physician complete current information concerning his diagnosis, treatment and prognosis in terms the patient can be reasonably expected to understand.* When it is not medically advisable to give such information to the patient the information should be made known to an appropriate person in his behalf. He has a right to know by name the physician responsible for his care. (our emphasis)

3. The patient has the right to receive from his physician information necessary to give informed consent prior to the start of any procedure and/or treatment. Except in emergencies, such information for informed consent should include but not necessarily be limited to the specific procedure or treatment, the medically significant risks involved and the probable duration of incapacitation. When medically significant alternatives for care or treatment exist, or when the patient requests information concerning medical alternatives, the patient has the right to such information. The patient also has the right to know the name of the person responsible for the procedures and/or treatment.

4. The patient has the right to refuse treatment to the extent permitted by law, and to be informed of the medical consequences of his action.

5. The patient has the right to every consideration of his privacy concerning his own medical care program. Case discussion, consultation, examination and treatment are confidential and should be conducted discreetly. Those not directly involved in his care must have the permission of the patient to be present.

6. The patient has the right to expect that all communications and records pertaining to his care should be treated as confidential.

7. The patient has the right to expect that within its capacity a hospital must make reasonable response to the request of a patient for services. The hospital must provide evaluation, service, and/or referral as indicated by the urgency of the case. When medically permissible a patient may be transferred to another facility only after he has received complete information and explanation concerning the needs for and alternatives to such a transfer. The institution to which the patient is to be transferred must first have accepted the patient for transfer.

8. The patient has the right to obtain information as to any relationship of his hospital to other health care and educational institutions insofar as his care is concerned. The patient has the right to obtain information as to the existence of any professional relationship between individuals, by name, who are treating him.

9. The patient has the right to be advised if the hospital proposes to engage in or perform human experimentation affecting his care and treatment. The patient has the right to refuse to participate in such research projects.

10. The patient has the right to expect reasonable continuity of care. He has the right to know in advance what appointment times and physicians are available and where. The patient has the right to expect that the hospital will provide a mechanism whereby he is informed by his physician or a delegate of the physician of the patient's continuing health care requirements following discharge.

11. The patient has the right to examine and receive an explanation of his bill, regardless of source of payment.

12. The patient has the right to know what hospital rules and regulations apply to his conduct as a patient. No catalog of rights can guarantee for the patient the kind of treatment he has a right to expect. A hospital has many functions to perform, including the prevention and treatment of disease, the education of both health professionals and patients, and the conduct of clinical research. All these activities must be conducted with an overriding concern for the patient, and, above all, the recognition of his dignity as a human being. Success in achieving this recognition assures success in the defense of the rights of the patient.

CHAPTER 4 ❈ *Before Surgery*

> *It's good to hope. It's the waiting that spoils it.*
> Yiddish proverb

There's no such thing as a typical waiting period before ostomy surgery. Sometimes, there's no wait at all. The victim of an auto accident may end up with a temporary colostomy, even before news of the crash is reported on the radio. In life-threatening situations—a woman with her bladder mangled in a car crash, or a young man with a ruptured intestine—full explanations must come after surgery. Although there's no time to explain, the news is good—the car crash victim and the young man are alive, not dead.

For others, waiting seems endless. A person who has ulcerative colitis may have had miserable months or years to get ready, while one drug after another and one treatment after another were tried. By the time surgery is finally scheduled, such patients are usually eager for the freedom it promises.

I had nine days—a weekend at home and a week in the hospital — to get used to the idea of a colostomy. It was a double adjustment—both to the coming surgery and to the unexpected cancer that made it necessary.

If I'd lived closer to the hospital, many of the tests and some of the other preparation might have been done before I was admitted, since I was basically healthy and didn't need the kind of building up which some people need after a siege of severe bowel disease.

That weekend was dizzy and out of focus. Besides packing things I didn't need, and watering water-logged plants while neglecting bone-dry ones, I phoned people, saw them, went out to dinner, wrote maudlin heart-in-the mouth letters (and a last will and testament), explaining what little I knew. Although I rattled off the words like a parrot, I still didn't believe them. Then, and for the week that followed, I was cushioned by a strange sense of unreality. Surely I was only a stand-in; all the things they were talking about were really going to happen to someone else.

Driving back to San Francisco with friends Sunday afternoon, I fought the odd sensation that one tire was probably going to come off the car. When we got to the city, we discovered that one tire had been slashed almost all the way through and was seriously out of alignment! They had it fixed before they returned. I felt a little less crazy.

"Come to the hospital Monday morning by eight," Dr. Wise had invited. "Without breakfast, and without coffee."

It was an omen, and a preview. All that first week in the hospital, meals would appear on time for a day or so; then I wouldn't get a tray at mealtime.

"My food didn't come."

"Sorry, doctor's orders—there's that test."

Out in the big world, great things were happening. Athletes were arriving in Montreal for the start of the Olympics on July 17. I turned my back on the pageantry on my neighbor's TV and wondered how soon I would be able to eat after surgery. That week, my horizons were on the narrow side.

What Dr. Wise had said when he set up this elaborate charade was, "We'd like to do a few more tests." That seemed the understatement of the year. Twice daily, the doctors made their rounds. Usually, their first visit was almost before the cock crowed in the morning, and then they'd pop in again, late in the afternoon. Dr. Reinker, my surgeon, was usually accompanied by the resident working with him, Dr. Banks, and by an intern barely two weeks out of medical school, who clasped his hands behind his back and looked as solemn as he could. Sometimes other doctors came along.

After each visit, they must have sprinted back to the doctor's small cubbyhole next to the nursing station to write up another three dozen orders for tests, familiar and unfamiliar, plus all the usual routine things—blood pressure, pulse, and temperature. Amazing that they could fit them all in.

The week before, the diagnosis had been made with the help of a sigmoidoscope. This is a rather rigid tube which, inserted into the large intestine via the anus, gives the doctor a fair view of the last 12 or 14 inches of the intestinal tract, the area where hemorrhoids (and most cancers) appear.

Now they wanted to look beyond that, and so an examination with a *colonoscope* was scheduled. This far more sophisticated instrument is soft and flexible and provides a view of the entire six feet of the colon, so well lighted that slides or movies can be taken if desired. (The colonoscope can also be used for minor colon surgery—removing a polyp, for instance.)

That was Tuesday. On Thursday, after a brief starvation diet and more laxatives and enemas than I cared for, I was introduced to *barium enemas* and *intravenous pyelograms*. The barium enema, which seemed to involve quarts of pale, pink plaster inserted through the anus, fills the colon and makes a shadow picture of its twistings and turnings, together with any irregularities. X-rays are taken at various points in the barium's journey.

To complete the map they were making of my interior, the IVP (intravenous pyelogram) involves a substance which is injected into the arm. This travels through the kidneys and the rest of the urinary tract, and makes the urinary tract show up clearly on an x-ray, highlighting any malfunction and showing where kidneys and bladder are in relation to the colon and other landmarks. This test is relatively comfortable except for a brief but fiery heat flash following the injection. For those few people who are allergic to the injected substance, other tests can be used to give the necessary information about the urinary tract.

With any gaps in time filled with an *electrocardiogram* (EKG or ECG) to check heart function, and with more blood and urine tests to show how well my liver, kidneys, and lungs were functioning, the tests were coming to an end. From them, the doctors had a fair idea of how well my body would withstand the inevitable shock of surgery.

Mechanical and lab tests were only part of the endless information-gathering process. Although I'd just had a complete physical in the weeks before the malignancy was discovered, this was a teaching hospital, so I gave my history to a seemingly endless stream of eager listeners. I told about my illnesses, allergies and life style. Since all the doctors and nurses who questioned me had slightly different points of view and asked different questions, it was not pure repetition, although some days it seemed like overkill, as doctors poked and palpated, listened with a stethoscope, tested reflexes. . . .

There were some visitors, many cards, letters, and calls. Since my friend Irv had come to visit me the night I arrived, and told me the important thing about his colostomy just by being there, alive and healthy, I didn't think of requesting a UOA visitor before surgery, though I might have welcomed one. Many patients, not knowing an Irv, are dubious about seeing anyone with an ostomy before surgery, although it can be very reassuring. Judy Greaves of Coos Bay, Oregon, suggests: "The pre-op patient, waiting for this unknown, mysterious thing to happen to him, is too blamed scared to consent to anything. . . . [But] the result will be less fear of the unknown, because the patient has seen an apparently 'normal' person doing things he has always done and looking like everyone else. A short, pleasant visit by this stranger he thought of as 'mutilated' can do wonders for his morale. . . ." It could have helped.

From Monday afternoon, when the doctors came in and saw me enjoying a cigarette, there was heavy pressure to cut out cigarettes, at least for the present. As they explained it, if I stopped smoking, even for a few days, the irritation and mucus production in my lungs would decrease, and I would have a better chance of sailing through surgery and the days after without lung problems.

Their arguments moved me, and I did cut down drastically—from two packs a day to two or three cigarettes a day! I was helped in this by the respiratory therapist who talked more about the heavy load surgery puts on the lungs and the blood stream. She brought me (on loan) an engaging toy with a serious purpose. This was an *incentive spirometer.* When I put the tube in my mouth and took a really deep breath, three bright cheerful blue balls would rise to the top of their respective plastic columns. The deeper and steadier the breath, the longer they would stay at the top. Do it every hour, she suggested, but I was fascinated by this simple proof of progress in breathing, and sometimes tucked in an extra session.

I think my three roommates, a fascinating and ever-changing group (since most of them were in for minor surgery), envied me my breathing toy. I was frankly jealous of their meals, as mine petered out to nothing. There was a last bland meal on Friday night—chicken broth, baked halibut, asparagus cuts, and orange cake with frosting—and thereafter only clear liquids.

On Saturday, when I began a clear liquid diet, it seemed as if they gave me a laxative every two hours. It wasn't really that often, but I'd definitely begun the intensive period of bowel "prep" which precedes surgery of the colon. To prevent post-operative infections, and to have a clear field for surgery, surgeons, nurses, and dietitians work together to clean out the bowel; their purpose is to have the entire colon as fresh and clean as if they'd turned the hose on it. Not only any remnants of feces, but also as many as possible of the bacteria (friendly and unfriendly) which usually live in the colon, must be removed. The measures employed seem somewhat drastic to the patient.

There is a progression from low residue diet to clear liquid, and there's an increasing concentration on laxatives and then enemas. The specifics of bowel prep vary from doctor to doctor, from hospital to hospital, and even from time to time. When I was getting ready for the barium enema, I'd had the dubious treat of bubble-gum flavored castor oil; a couple of months later, when I had another barium enema as a postoperative check, it had been replaced by something slightly less revolting.

On the day before surgery, according to a brief note I made, I had a laxative, five enemas, and three showers! These were not the relatively simple do-it-yourself Fleets prepackaged enemas, but the old-fashioned kind, administered by a determined nurse. In addition, just in case any bacteria escaped this all-out onslaught, there were antibiotics.

The Saturday and Sunday before surgery were marked by other highlights. People kept coming in and introducing themselves. "Hi, I'm one of the recovery-room nurses, so you'll recognize a familiar face when you wake up in the recovery room." "Hello, I'm the anesthetist, and I wonder if you have any questions."

The day before surgery, Dr. Reinker took me into his office, explained just what they would be doing, and, after considering my body sitting, standing, and lying, marked the probable site of the stoma with a brown felt-tip pen. In some hospitals, an ET would have done this, or at least participated.

I was overcome by strange longings, almost like those of pregnancy. In the middle of that endless day, with nothing but clear liquids sloshing around in me, I spotted Dr. Banks and made a solemn request. If my daughter would just bring me some salted soda crackers, could I lick the salt off them? We had an earnest discussion of this important though silly question. Finally, he decided he could trust me not to swallow a crumb and agreed, giving me a hug as he did so.

Though there was no time wasted on meals that last day, it was busy, between all the enemas and the three showers. I've never quite understood the rationale for those!

There'd been unmentioned highlights all week long, together with my complaining. My daughter Kerry and my son-in-law Art came in often, though I couldn't have chosen a worse week for them, given their hectic schedules. Michael Wise, the doctor who'd found the cancer, slipped in frequently, just to talk a little.

I'd brought *Walden* along, thinking I might share some beautiful thoughts with Henry David Thoreau that week, but usually I was mired thigh-deep in trivia. Still, it was a comfort to know I had a good book with me, should I need it.

And if I'd opened it, I might have chuckled at passages like this, curiously appropriate to the last day before surgery: "Simplify, simplify. Instead of three meals a day, if it be necessary eat but one; instead of a hundred dishes, five; and reduce other things in proportion."

That might have been a good thought while drifting off to sleep, following the fairly heavy sedative Sunday night. That or: "...what danger is there if you don't think of any?"

CHAPTER 5

Surgery, and Just After

Recovery room nurses are used to receiving a lot of flak from woozy patients—and abject apologies a week or two later. . . .

Some ostomates are old pros at post-surgical rituals. I was a novice, a reluctant and even faintly belligerent newcomer to the aftermath of abdominal surgery. In theory, I might still be a member of my treatment team; in practice, I was on the bench for a time.

The last thing I remember, after the pre-op shots and the journey to the operating room on a rolling stretcher, was lecturing a masked figure in green who was shaving my lower abdomen in some surgical anteroom.

"Why did you wait till the last minute?" I asked, a little fuzzily. "When I had toe surgery [twenty-five years before], they shaved my leg the night before—all the way to the hip, painted it with Merthiolate, and then wrapped it in a pillowcase so it wouldn't get dirty."

"We do it here in the surgical area right before the operation to decrease the number of skin bacteria."

How clever, I thought, and fell asleep.

The next thing I remember was waking up in the recovery room, hours after surgery.

Now lovely chunks of sleep were interrupted by torture. Someone—a nurse I supposed—kept waking me up.

"Take a deep breath and cough."

"I can't."

"Yes, you can. Breathe deep now, and cough."

She seemed not only mean but stupid. Didn't she know that sleep is the great healer? That sleep knits up the raveled sleeve of care?

If only they'd stop nagging and leave me alone! I'd nod off and then another voice would cut in, "Come on, now, you have to take a deep breath and cough."

Yet—underneath this running battle with the nurses—an odd awareness surfaced from time to time. For better or for worse, surgery was over. And I was alive. It wasn't a constant thought— but it was magic when it came.

There are, I discovered, good reasons for those painful and seemingly endless commands during the first few days after surgery—*take a deep breath* and *cough*. Among other things, they help prevent lung complications.

No one longs for the not-so-good old days when a bullet to bite on and a jigger of rum sustained people through surgery. General anesthesia—which makes possible deep unconsciousness during an operation—has revolutionized surgery. However, anesthetics make great demands on the body, especially the lungs. Anesthetics irritate the lining of the lungs; these, in response, produce extra mucus to soothe the irritation. The anesthetic also paralyzes the tiny hairs in the respiratory tract which normally sweep mucus out of the lungs. If the mucus isn't removed, it clogs the air sacs in the lungs so they can't inflate with air. The temporarily collapsed air sacs become warm, moist havens for bacteria.

Energetic and frequent coughing and deep breathing help loosen and bring up mucus so the airway remains free. Coughing is more comfortable if a patient hugs a pillow or two tightly over the abdominal incision. This splints the wound and reduces the fear that the stitches will pop open. They won't, even without a pillow.

As some doctors do, mine kept me in the recovery room overnight. It was quieter there than on the ward, with more nurses available for the almost constant monitoring, and special equipment, should it be needed.

In the recovery room, extra oxygen is frequently given as a routine aid to the lungs after anesthesia; the presence of an oxygen tank doesn't mean an emergency. Electrodes on the chest, hooked up by wires to a heart monitor, trace the heart's activity on a screen. Again, this is usually a routine precaution, not a sign of crisis. (Some hospitals encourage people waiting for surgery to visit the recovery room before the operation so they'll know what to expect.)

When I was returned to my room the next morning, I was introduced to new forms of misery.

"Welcome back, Mrs. Mullen. How are you feeling?"

I didn't answer.

"It's time to walk now."

Walk! They were out of their minds. It hurt too much just to turn over in bed. But I walked, lurching and hurting.

It was a nurse, John, who taught me the secret of moving with less pain. "OK, now, before you try to turn over, take a deep breath and let it out slowly as you turn. You can't tense your muscles while you're expelling your breath." Absurd and simple-minded though his remedy sounded, it worked, not only for turning over but for getting out of bed. And walking.

As it turns out, there are excellent reasons for walking, as for coughing. Lying in bed too long can cause problems after surgery. When people lie down, their lungs don't expand as well as they do when they stand or walk. In addition, blood tends to slow down on its return to the heart, and may form small clots. To prevent these and other bad effects of prolonged bedrest, patients walk, willingly or unwillingly.

I'd been so busy defending myself against all these orders that I hadn't paid much attention to my new status as a porcupine. Back in my room, I saw that there was a tube in my hand, another in my nose, and one going to the bladder. Each tube was attached to something on the outside.

I'd expected the IV, for I'd had one before. This tube, inserted directly into a vein, serves as a life-line, making possible the swift administration of blood, fluids, medicines, and anesthetics. The IV tube is connected to plastic pouches or a glass bottle, filled with fluids, fastened on a portable stand. From a patient's viewpoint, the IV has great nuisance value. If I walked, it went along.

I had not expected the tube which went through my nose and down the esophagus to the stomach. As a rule, the intestinal tract goes into hibernation for a few days after abdominal surgery. Until the intestines start working again, this tube, called a nasogastric or NG tube, is connected to a suction machine to remove gas and stomach secretions. Without the help of this small tube, these would build up and cause acute discomfort and vomiting. Sore throats, a common complaint after any major surgery, are more often caused by another tube, this one inserted after the person is asleep in the operating room and removed before the person wakes up, to deliver the long-lasting anesthetic through the mouth and into the lungs, and to make breathing easier during the operation.

Finally, there was a catheter or tube inserted directly into the bladder to drain urine into an external bag. The bladder, inevitably pushed around some during abdominal surgery, may turn sluggish for a time. The external collection bag allows staff to check the urine output. It's also convenient not to have to worry about wet beds or coping with a bedpan when sitting and moving are still such a painful, risky business.

So, when I walked I had company: the IV stand, the NG tube and the somewhat embarrassing bag full of urine. No one paid any attention.

Like many new ostomates, I was in no hurry to survey the

alterations to my anatomy. Since the digestive system has slowed to a halt, the person with an ileostomy or a colostomy can ignore the stoma for a few days after surgery. One sneaks a look—it is there, red and foreign, inside the plastic post-op appliance, but it isn't doing much and it doesn't hurt.

The incision does hurt. There's a glimpse of that, too, when the dressing is changed. For most colostomates and many ileostomates, the most painful sensations come from a wound one can't see—the large opening where the rectum and anus used to be. This wound—which will make sitting difficult for weeks to come—is treated in different ways by different surgeons.

The urostomate, on the other hand, cannot ignore the new stoma. With the bladder removed and disconnected, urine discharge is constant, from the minute the stoma is constructed on the operating table. Urostomates are spared the bladder catheter, and retain rectum and anus so they don't have that rear wound.

I tried to catch up.

"Why didn't the doctor come and see me in the recovery room after surgery?" I asked my daughter.

"He did—three times. Doctor Wise came too. And so did I."

"Really? That's nice." I said it as politely as I could, knowing that she was kidding me. If they'd come, surely I would have remembered?

But maybe not. There was a big blank spot when I couldn't have remembered if a bagpipe corps had come and serenaded me (that would have been nice). The memory blank results from the aftereffects of anesthesia, fairly heavy pain and sleep medication in the first few days after surgery, and perhaps the body's intuitive need to protect itself from pain.

I think I asked the same questions dozens of times.

"How long was I in surgery?"

"About four hours."

"Did I have any transfusions?"

"Yes, four units of blood."

"The tumor—was it really malignant?"

"Yes."

"Did you get it all?"

"We hope so."

Every ostomate has a different experience in surgery. More important, everyone reacts differently. We differ in our tolerance for pain and/or discomfort, the speed with which we heal, the swiftness with which we wake up after surgery, and many other things. And though some patterns may seem luckier than others, no one way is right. . . .

In spite of my grumbles, I was lucky. Thanks to those nagging nurses (and a basically healthy body), there were no post-op complications except the minor bladder infection which sometimes follows catherization of the bladder. And people had come to see me, even if I didn't remember them.

For most patients, the days just after surgery tend to be foggy, thanks to the anesthetic, continuing pain medication, and both body and mind's resistance to change. One is not always rational or logical. Still, with much help from nursing staff, family and friends, most of us manage to muddle through.

The surgery had taken place Monday morning. On Thursday, the doctor was delighted when my system started a noisy rumbling. That meant my body was beginning to take over its own chores again, and so the NG tube could go. I could eat and drink, even though that first meal—apple juice, chicken broth, and lemon jello—was not much of a reward.

But I was alive. Alive and beginning to hope.

So—when I ran into the recovery-room nurse waiting for the elevator, I apologized for calling her a bitch.

CHAPTER 6 ✤ *On the Mend*

Learn the lines and get on with it.
Spencer Tracy

With the tubes out, medication cut down, and solid food promised (if not yet delivered), it was time to open my eyes and really look at the changes surgery had made.

It would also have been a good time to remember the Serenity Prayer, but I'm not sure that I did:

SERENITY PRAYER

God grant me the serenity to accept
the things I cannot change,
the courage to change the things I can,
and the wisdom to know the difference.

At the time, my biggest problem was that last line, "the wisdom to know the difference." One of these days, surely, everything would be put back together the way it was supposed to be?

In a more realistic mood, I realized I couldn't change the stoma, but I could get acquainted with it, perhaps teach it manners, or even show it who was boss.

I couldn't change the wound where my rectum and anus used to be; however—back now to a normal diet and a little more exercise —perhaps I could speed its healing.

The next day, we moved to a larger and warmer bathroom, and they brought a real colostomy irrigating set with a small, smooth, cone-shaped piece of plastic to fit over the end of the irrigating tube; but the experience still wasn't a happy one.

"Tell you what," said the doctor, "we'll get Jean Alvers to come over and show you how to do it. She's an ET."

Jean came that night and I was cheered by her visit. She explained some of the hows and whys of irrigating. The next morning, I told the nurses I would do it myself, and I did. It was a success, but I still didn't like the process, or want to repeat it.

Irrigation is a happy choice for thousands of colostomates. For others, including me, it is not. A strong dislike for enemas in any form (a souvenir of my childhood) had been reinforced by the bowel prep the week before surgery, and by those frustrating first attempts.

By then, I'd had a visitor from Golden Gate Chapter of the United Ostomy Association, and she'd left me a treasure of a booklet: *Colostomies — A Guide.* Somewhere in the middle, I found this sentence: "Some people with a descending or a sigmoid colostomy find that by eating selected foods at specific intervals, they can make the bowel move at a time convenient to them."

From that day on, whenever the doctor asked about irrigation, I shook my head and showed him the book. He was, I think, a little baffled by my stubbornness, but he did say, "It's your decision."

For an appliance, I discovered by chance a makeshift one which worked reasonably well; if it was something less than ideal, at least the management of my stoma was in my own hands.

Jean Alvers had left her phone number and had encouraged me to call if there were any problems, but I hesitated to bother her. That was a mistake. If I had called, I might have learned about other secure alternatives much sooner. Those first days are the time to learn the rudiments of control: skin care, appliance choice, emptying, changing, cleaning, and all the other rituals of this new life. Many ostomates may need or wish to change materials and methods later. The important thing in the hospital is to learn a reasonably comfortable way to deal with one's stoma and be able to do it independently by the time of discharge (barring other physical problems which may make help necessary, at least temporarily).

The doctors continued their twice daily rounds, admiring the stoma and checking the incision. It was a beautiful stoma, the surgeon insisted. Although beautiful was not the word I would have chosen, I later discovered that it is indeed an excellent stoma, neat and of a good size.

At first, I found the doctors' constant interest in the gaping wound between my buttocks curious and mildly embarrassing, but one adjusts. And they were paying attention where it seemed appropriate. My biggest discomfort remained that pain in my butt — the *perineal* or *posterior wound*. It felt bruised; it was impossible to sit squarely on it. It was less pain than acute discomfort—the kind of sore, aching numbness that sometimes happens after horseback riding, without any of the pleasure.

Most colostomates and many ileostomates have such a wound where the rectum and anus used to be, and a most peculiar wound it is. In many operations, when surgeons remove an organ, they can count on other nearby organs to fill in the cavity. Not so when rectum and anus are removed. Because of the bony structures surrounding the area, no other organs can move into the gap.

What the body does—at varying rates of speed—is to form scar tissue to fill this hole.

Surgeons have different techniques for dealing with the empty space in the meantime. Some simply leave the wound open, packing it firmly with gauze. As the wound heals from the inside out, the space gets smaller and smaller and the amount of gauze is reduced.

Other surgeons loosely baste the skin together, inserting soft drainage tubes to remove blood and other fluid by gravity. This was the treatment I had; soft, thick, absorbent pads were fastened loosely over the area with paper tape (a rather casual approach, it seemed to me). Drainage, heavy at first, tapers off so that smaller pads can be used.

In another alternative, tubes from the wound are attached to a suction device. This removes fluids and may help the wound to close sooner without complications.

Whatever the technique, it takes time for the body to create the scar tissue to fill that empty space.

Perineal wounds are mysterious in many ways. Some heal in two months or less. Others (though drainage and discomfort have decreased) may take a year or more.

The day after the doctor ordered three sitz baths a day for me, I wanted to hug him. Basically, a sitz bath involves sitting for 15 or 20 minutes three times a day in about six inches of very warm water. The heat eases soreness and relaxes muscles. It also increases blood circulation to the area, speeding healing.

My hospital had built-in sitz baths in special small rooms. The baths resemble large wash tubs, but they're installed at floor level and gleam with white enamel. At home, one can improvise with a large plastic tub or a generous-sized baby bath tub. A full tub bath doesn't work as well, since soaking in a full bath 20 minutes three times a day drains away too much energy. In the hospital or at home, a thick folded bath towel on the bottom of sitz bath or tub makes sitting easier.

Some doctors now recommend that new ostomates use a dental irrigating device to clean the wound and help it heal faster.

In the hospital, I learned to carry a bed pillow with me, wherever I walked, just in case I decided to sit down. Even then, I sat gingerly, on one buttock or the other. A square of foam rubber, three to four inches thick, makes a good portable seat. Doughnut-shaped inflated rings should not be used, since they can encourage the wound to pull apart.

Sensations in the perineal wound or the area around it differ. Many report a continuing urge to defecate in the old way; this sensation is comparable to the "phantom limb" sensation, common to amputees. Although the necessary equipment is missing, the nerves are still active. The sensation usually diminishes with time.

There are also aching and tingling sensations; these also decrease as healing proceeds. If problems of pain, drainage, or infection continue, it's time to consult a doctor.

For the new ostomate, the days in the hospital after surgery are busy, even crowded. There is so much to learn, so many different things to try to cope with. There are also decisions to make—or at least consider.

Not long before I went home, Dr. Reinker and I talked some about the malignancy that had brought all this about. He hoped they had gotten every last cancer cell, but there had been some spread. The cancer was in several adjoining lymph nodes so these had been removed; with luck, no stray cells would be wandering around the lymphatic system.

He recommended that I consider a course of radiation, aimed at the perineal area, as a precautionary measure. The consulting doctors agreed. However, the decision did not have to be made at once, and, he emphasized, it would be my decision.

As I remember, I was so absorbed with the day-to-day details of dealing with the stoma, comforting the perineal area with sitz baths and soft cushions, and trying to move back to reality (wherever that might be), that the word *cancer* didn't really register with me. And yet I'm sure it was there, in my unconscious. At that time, I knew two colostomates. My friend Irv, whose ostomy was temporary, was doing fine; my friend Susan was not. She'd had surgery many weeks before I had; when I was discharged and went home, Susan was still in the hospital, and still in bed most of the time. It was scary to wonder which path I might follow.

I was supposed to be resting, taking it easy, and yet there were all these problems to face, or postpone facing. I could echo what actress Barbara Bel Geddes said of her own mastectomy: "There's no sense in saying it's a little itty, bitty thing. It was a helluva blow."

The mail brought welcome though sometimes puzzling cards

and letters from friends. Helen wrote, "If anybody was prepared for what you are going through, it is you. And I'm proud of you, gal."

Prepared? How?

Proud? Why?

Although energy was returning, it was still in short supply. Relatively minor nuisances loomed like major plagues. Like many people, I developed a bladder infection as a result of the bladder catheter; this causes a desire to urinate almost constantly and a burning sensation. Fever may also be a symptom. Antibiotics and plenty of fluids are the usual treatment.

Although I sometimes wondered at her patience with my vapors, my daughter continued to be a frequent and welcome visitor. Sometimes my son-in-law or a grandchild came along. Friends and relatives cheered me with short visits, and I enjoyed talking with my roommates as well as doctors and nurses.

Small things delighted me. The hospital had a short supply of soft, old, much-laundered gowns, and a big supply of new and stiff ones. It was a good day when a friendly nurse slipped me a soft one.

Along with mastering the here and now, there has to be some planning for the future. Here the social worker may be a resource, as well as the discharge planning team at the hospital. When finances are critical, they will know what may be available in the way of aid. Government disability payments now come through the Social Security Administration. To receive them, one must be either totally disabled or expect to be disabled for at least one year. Most ostomates simply do not qualify—they'll be up and about long before a year has passed. Emergency funds may be available through General Assistance, and the ostomate may qualify for Medicaid (MediCal in California).

I was ambivalent about leaving the hospital, in spite of what they'd done to me. It would be great to be home again, and yet part of me savored that sheltered existence, where other people made many of the decisions—or at least did the leg work.

And—one mystery remained.

When I'd started the physical which led to finding the cancer which led to the surgery which led to the colostomy, I'd been 100% sure that I had a stomach ulcer.

Where had it gone?

CHAPTER 7 But How Do You Really Feel?

In the weeks after surgery, trifles seemed to bother me most—small woes standing in for bigger ones I wasn't ready to face. When the diet kitchen didn't send my milk, I swiveled into a rage. If the vending machine in the hospital canteen grabbed my quarters, giving nothing in return, I was awash with tears. And yet, when Dr. Wise asked, "How do you really feel?" I chirped "Fine!" Sometimes I was lying. . . .

Of course positive thinking has great value, many clouds have silver linings, and we should all look at the bright side of things.

But trying to rush the Pollyanna process seldom works. We can't even see the bright side until we've allowed ourselves to really feel our sorrow. Our sorrow. Our anger. Our sense of loss. And our fear.

However we may try to kid ourselves, for most ostomates there's bound to be a sense of outrage when we glimpse our changed body, and also a nostalgic longing for the way things used to be, before all of this happened. Though our bowels or our bladders may have caused us pain, embarrassment, trouble, and even isolation for weeks or months or years, we were used to them. They were part of us, long taken for granted systems which had provided us with simple but constant satisfaction for more years than we could remember. Tattered and worn though the afflicted portions of our intestines or our bladders might have been, they were ours.

And now they are gone.

As Richard J. Wells, M.D. said: "People still have an inordinate emotional attachment to their own organs of elimination no matter how diseased they become. They will gladly part with a gall bladder, a stomach, 90% of their liver, or even a piece of brain, but suggest removing the bladder or the rectum and the red lights begin to blink."

Sometimes that grief is irrational — a person with ulcerative colitis doesn't lose control with surgery but regains it — yet that doesn't make the sorrow any smaller. We're not always rational people. However wise and grownup we've managed to become, there's a shadow of a hurt child underneath.

But things aren't the way they used to be, and we have stomas to prove it. And that is sorrow number two. There was a reasonably nice, reasonably slender abdomen and now there's a puffy lump with an incision, plus that *thing*, all veiled in plastic. It's true the incision is healing, the puffiness is receding, and I'm long past the age for entering the Miss America contest, but still — I had this image of myself, and now it's changed.

There is also a new vocabulary. People from many cultures have been taught to be silent — at least in polite society — about excretory functions. Thus, ostomates may wince at this new necessity of calling a spade a spade, of using blunt words like *feces* and *rectum* and *anus* instead of "the little girl's room."

There's something else. We're different now, different from most people we know. And we don't like that. Growing up, we wanted a doll like Sarah's or a bike like Jim's, and later, a car like Peter's and a house like the Smiths'. It was safer, not being different, but now we are.

That's a lot of sorrows. If we pretend they're not there, they're apt to fester and grow. However, let out of hiding, our grief and sorrow seem to run their course and dwindle down to a manageable size, so we can begin to savor life again, including the surgery which gave us a second chance. We even begin to see the funny side—sometimes.

But just as we're not always completely rational, we're not always completely honest. And there are temptations. We want medals for bravery (since we can no longer win them for going potty!) and so we lie.

"How do you feel?"

"Fine and dandy."

Only we don't. We're just putting on (or trying to put on) shining faces for staff and visitors—especially family—and for ourselves. Postponing the mourning—the good cry that's a necessary step in healing. Only after tears can the funny bone be operative again.

There's also a strange and ironic emotional peekaboo in trying too hard to be brave. Close relatives and friends were also grieving —about me and for me. Their feelings were different than mine, perhaps, but no less strong: "We were sad about the changes that had happened to you and, like you, angry at whatever fate made this surgery necessary. We wanted to reach out and let you know how much we cared. Sometimes we could. Other days, you pushed us away with your smile, your jaunty reassurance that everything was fine."

Shared laughter grows but shared grief tends to shrink, exposed to air and sun. If others are grieving with you, don't work too hard to hide your tears, or force them to postpone theirs.

It's a curious thing. We don't have to recount all these sorrows to everyone, and maybe not to anyone but ourselves. What we must do, though, is recognize them. Then, though traces of sadness may continue to surface from time to time, we don't have to cry very long. I remember with thanks a nurse who not only permitted me to cry through her lunch but encouraged me to do so.

As Victor Alter, RN, ET, wrote in the *ET Journal*. "What the new ostomate must begin to do then is to let go: let go of his former body image; let go of his diseased bladder or bowel; let go of the secondary gains that often accompany illness; in short, let go of all those feelings, thoughts and memories that keep him from becoming the person he is now. . . .

"It often happens that a new ostomate cannot begin this process of letting go and freeing himself. Sometimes just thinking about all that has happened is too awful. The person appears to be in despair, and despair colors the way one looks at all of reality. It is the patient's view of reality that needs scrutiny."

Looking back, I may have tried a little too hard to sidestep this process of mourning. A more honest look at how I felt in those weeks just after surgery might have prevented some black periods. later.

And yet, although this necessary process of mourning these changes cannot be evaded, neither can it be pushed and hurried. Each of us brings different weaknesses—and strengths—to this encounter with reality, and a certain innate mind-body wisdom may control the timing of the confrontation.

Gertrud Ujhely, RN, says: ". . . the danger of grief does not lie in what one feels, but rather in one's inability to tolerate one's experience . . . one's blocking or repressing one's state . . . the feelings, whether accepted or not, continue to lead their own existence—if necessary, outside one's awareness."

For all of us who have ostomies because a malignancy has been discovered, there is a double-header of shock, sorrow, and fear. Cancer is still one of the big scare words, hard to accept as having any personal meaning for us. I suspect some of us spend an inordinate amount of time fussing about our stomas so we won't have a chance to look at the other—and darker—side of the coin: "Did they get it all?" "How long do I have?" "What's the use?"

Such determined pessimism doesn't leave enough room for sensible optimism and determination. Great strides have been and continue to be made in the war against cancer. With early detection, there's a reasonable chance that they did get it all.

There are also still too many unknowns about "cancer," which is not just one disease but a catch-all term for more than 100 disorders! These range from some which grow very slowly to others which spread quickly.

And—there's the mysterious factor of remission. For reasons no one understands, the six months that were all a doctor could promise have a way of stretching.

When Elsie Klein of Pennsylvania was 76, a busy widow managing her own home and large garden, she noticed a change in her bowel habits. After many tests, the doctors discovered she had well-advanced cancer of the rectum. It had spread into her reproductive organs, requiring not only a colostomy but also a hysterectomy.

Her surgery was hard and convalescence slow. The doctor could promise no more than six months. An excellent seamstress, she proceeded to design and make her own "funeral dress," and made other arrangements. Once she'd done what she had to, she got busy living for the present—concentrating on her flower garden, making two huge hooked rugs, getting involved with other projects and with people.

The six months passed quickly. So did one year, two, three. . . . Six years after her surgery, her surgeon died.

On September 24, 1979, Elsie Klein celebrated her 92nd birthday, still happy and alert. The "funeral dress" is still waiting for her, 16 years after surgery. She smiles when asked about the dress. "It's probably yellowed with age."

Wynn Bullock, the famous photographer, didn't go along with the idea of cancer in his future after his colostomy. When his doctor said he had only six months to live, Bullock answered, "I have too many things to do to die that soon!" He proceeded to finish some important writing projects, take a few more photographs, star in a movie about his photography, and work his way through a huge stack of projects for the next two years!

His widow, Edna Bullock, remembers that he said, "Well, having cancer, what do I want to do? Do I want to sit around and think about it? I want to think about things I'm interested in. . . . Everything we do now is constructive, and it will continue to be."

Feelings of outrage, sorrow, fear and anger are normal and getting through them — or most of them — is a necessary chore. Many ostomates I've talked to agree that once in a while, there may be a brief tweak of old sorrow popping up, even five or 10 years later. By that time, though, so many new good things have happened that the memory is usually briefer than a quick sprinkle of rain.

Some people start to take an honest look at their feelings and then are so paralyzed they don't move on through to the other side, the good side. That's really sad — when people can't see the wide horizon beyond their ostomies.

Victor Alter concludes, "In the long run, the rehabilitation of the ostomy patient will not depend on whether his appliance is vinyl or rubber, belted or beltless, clear or opaque. The ostomate who accepts himself, the one who has resolved his loss successfully, will be capable of meeting his appliance needs.

"The ostomate who still feels empty, depressed, angry, and ashamed, whose energy is spent trying to contain those memories from which he cannot separate himself, may not only have appliance problems, but also other physical symptoms that result from repressing so many strong feelings of loss."

Neither ETs, nurses, nor doctors have unlimited time for listening and counseling, much as they may wish for elastic days. The ostomate who does not begin to glimpse a rainbow after a month or two might consider a brief course of professional counseling — at a mental health clinic or with a psychiatrist or other therapist who understands the many complexities and mysteries of adjusting to bodily change. After all, a second chance at life is too big a bonus to waste or fritter away with worry and gloom.

CHAPTER 8 ❄ *That Strange Big World Out There*

Although one me was eager to get out of the hospital, all the other me's were terrified at the idea, and it was the cowards who had a quorum. . . .

Four weeks and two days before, the hospital and all the things they were talking about doing to me there had seemed unreal. Now, everything was topsy-turvy. It was the "real" world that seemed strange and unreal, and the hospital which seemed real. Of course that feeling, like many others that would surface in the next few months, was transient.

When I was discharged, I camped with my daughter and her family in their home near the hospital, until they took off on a long-planned vacation (and my check-ups stretched out to once a week). While there I slept a lot, worried some, and made a few timid trips to the store. Then my cousin and his wife drove me back home to Santa Rosa, with a thoughtful stop at the supermarket to stock up on all the things my empty apartment wouldn't have.

A day or two later, I wrote to a friend: "With the wound healing, I can sit better and am having small but steady quantum leaps of energy. Yesterday, friends came over and fixed dinner, washed the dishes, vacuumed but talked too late.

"I've not yet adjusted to here—forget where things are and what kind of coffee cups I have. . . ."

If I didn't know what kind of coffee cups I had, who did? Divorced for a number of years, I was used to living alone and enjoyed many parts of such a life. The process of getting back into the world again would be much different if there were a spouse waiting—possibly better, possibly worse, but certainly different.

There were good friends close by in the apartment complex who welcomed me back, yet I felt lonely after the hospital. In part, at least, this was a communication problem. I didn't want to think about my colostomy all the time (and there were longer and longer periods when I forgot all about it), but it still had a way of creeping into my mind, wanted or not.

Sometimes, with a private chuckle, I'd hear an expression like "get your shit together" and find it all too apt (had that vulgarity been coined by an ostomate?). Or I would be reminded, for instance, as I figured out that the small paper-like fragments in my stool were not parchment but potato skins! In the hospital, a roommate, a nurse or a doctor would have shared the joke. However, I doubted whether any of my neighbors would be amused by such an early-morning confidence!

In a way, the joke was on me. I'd always thought discussions about bowel habits an extra-large bore and had avoided them when I could. With so many fascinating things in the world to talk about, how could anyone want to waste time talking about the virtues of a new laxative? Or share their anxiety because they couldn't get "regular?" The worst, just a few weeks before, had been someone who'd discovered the joys of coffee enemas!

And now here I was, often finding the activities of my digestive system the most fascinating topic in the world! The United Ostomy Association came to my rescue. In answer to my call, I had not one but two visitors, pronto. Ann Kaufman and Dorothy Siercks were all the things UOA visitors should be, including lots of fun (and we've been good friends ever since). Because they shared my amusement at the strange ways of stomas (not to mention their owners), the colostomy could begin to move away from center stage.

It didn't take long to find out that Ann and Dorothy were both interested in a great many things besides ostomies. Ann and her husband Ed are excellent sailors and Ann sparkled like sun on the water when she told about a recent day's sailing on San Francisco Bay. Dorothy and her husband, Lloyd, are tireless weekend explorers, fishing and camping all over Northern California.

When my visitors left, they gave me a wonderful stack of back issues of *Ostomy Quarterly,* the official publication of the United Ostomy Association. Even though I was plumb in the middle of an exciting mystery novel, it got shoved aside that night. Here, perhaps, were some of the answers I'd been looking for. It was good to find such an interesting group of people, thinking about some of the same big problems that worried me, and fretting about some of the same little ones.

In addition to the boost I got from Ann's and Dorothy's visit, subsequent phone calls, and UOA meetings I began to attend, the mail brought many unexpected shots in the arm, letters from old friends and letters from strangers. That happened this way. For the past two years, I'd been writing a light-hearted column for a local weekly, the *Santa Rosa News Herald.* When David Bolling, the editor, wrote and asked: "What's it like? Painful? Inconvenient? Frustrating? Frightening? . . . What causes rectal cancer? Please don't read that as the mercenary musings of an editor incapable of talking about real life. I'm curious, vicariously afraid. . . . What the hell? Drop me some notes."

Although I was timid about giving my neighbor, Mrs. Jones, a play-by-play account of my surgery, I decided to write a relatively light-hearted column about the adventure. The response was great — letters, phone calls, even requests for help (as if six or seven weeks of trial and error made me some kind of an expert).

An old friend, Marian, wrote, "What's the big deal? My

mother has had her colostomy for 17 years now, and it's never slowed her down." Remembering Marian's mother, I knew that.

A writer I knew surprised me with this note, showing an awareness of both the downs and the ups:

I have a close awareness of a colostomy, as I nursed my mother through her post surgery with the same procedure. She, like yourself, had tremendous spirit and determination and rose above even that. When you are sharing daily a problem such as this, you realize all the ramifications.

Also, I have another friend who is in her forties who has had an ileostomy. She was the one who encouraged me to go to the singles dances when I was widowed. We'd dress up, get in her truck, away we'd go to the St. Francis, dance half the night, compare notes after, while eating ham and eggs at Denny's. She always was the belle of the ball and had more boy friends than she could tuck away. On top of that, she decided she wanted to learn professional hair styling and went to beauty college along with all the bubble-headed teenagers. Got her license and opened her own shop.

In addition to sharing true life stories, the mail brought good suggestions, some from people who had had ostomies, but more from people who had had other major surgery. They all warned me about the same thing—fatigue—and though I knew about that intellectually, I couldn't seem to remember it in practice. Any major surgery, especially abdominal surgery, slows one down. As I wrote to one of them: "Yes, impatience is the enemy. My surgery was two months ago yesterday and everyone, including the surgeon, thinks I'm getting along great, but there are times when I wonder. Part of my problem is feeling too good, relatively, so that about every other day I manage to overdo and then spend the next day catching up."

Phyllis had had a mastectomy and she said, "Be prepared to go into a wingding every time you feel an odd twinge. We become cowards and die a thousand deaths. First you're sure it's your brain (that's an easy one) or what was that sudden pain under the rib?

You coughed! MY GOD. So if you can swing with all those little devils of metastasis, you've really got it made—but *do* get plenty of rest."

Even with that big headline, "A Colostomy," on my newspaper column, people could still wish me well—and ignore the details. "You're up and around?" "Oh yes. I had a bit of abdominal surgery and now I'm feeling better every day." "Good."

There's a lot of trial and error along the way, but walking gets easier, as do eating, and staying up really late (like until ten o'clock!).

Part of the trick is that the energy to move comes from moving; on the other hand, the longer one stays in bed, the longer one stays in bed. It may take a month or two for even the most proper digestive system to get back to normal. A lot of the problems are in the head. If you think you're sick, it's harder to get well than if you think you're getting well (and after all, you survived spareribs and sauerkraut last night, so maybe it's true).

Some anonymous UOA member wrote, "Learning to live with the new ostomy may be a satisfactory adjustment, but it is not the best. It is better to decide that it is going to have to live with you in the kind of life you want to live. Surprisingly, if you truly mean it, the ostomy will be quite co-operative. The best adjustment I have seen is the patient who said quite sincerely, 'If God had stopped to think a bit, He would have put them on the abdomen to begin with.'"

If a parent of a young child has an ostomy, the most important part of the explanation is the reassurance that now Mom (or Dad or whoever) will be healthier. When a parent is ill or hospitalized, children often are terrified; they need to know that they are not in any way to blame. The physical explanations can be very simple. An ostomy is just a different place for the bowel movement or urine to come out of the body. This was necessary to make the parent healthy again.

Children are curious and may want to see appliances or the stoma. Ostomates can respond in whatever way they feel comfortable. In any case, openness and matter-of-factness are the best approaches. Children frequently surprise us with the maturity and caring of their responses.

Children's questions can't be shrugged off or avoided. My grandchildren were beyond the toddler stage, so Kerry took over the questions and answers before I got home from the hospital.

"Were they curious?" I asked the other day.

"They still are—curious and quite supportive."

"How so?"

"Well, like Steve offered to do the drawings for *The Ostomy Book*. I told him two co-authors from one family were enough!"

CHAPTER 9 ❧ *Colostomies:*
Changes and Choices

People have one thing in common; they are all different.
Robert Zend

Colostomies are the oldest of the ostomies. The first ones —
pretty much trial and error — were done about the time of the
American Revolution and shortly thereafter. Nineteenth century
medical journals bristled with debates about how, why, when, and
where such surgery — first called a *preternatural anus* and later an
artificial anus — should be performed. For a time, lumbar
colostomies were favored, although it's hard to imagine how
anyone managed a stoma located on the lower back. Since, with
some exceptions, a colostomate's life expectancy wasn't very
promising at that time, perhaps no one worried about how the
patient would take care of the colostomy.

By the latter part of the 19th century, colostomies were
becoming more common, but there were still difficulties — both
in doing the surgery and in surviving it. And yet, the body has
such a strong will to survive, it often does, against very long odds.
In 1968, the *Ostomy Quarterly* had a feature about Miss Miriam
Coney, who'd had her colostomy in 1884 at the age of 20. She

survived eight brothers and sisters to celebrate 84 years with a colostomy *and* her 104th birthday in 1968!

The year 1908 was a turning point, when William Ernest Miles, M.D., performed the first abdomino-perineal resection of the rectum for cancer. Since the body must have a constantly available exit for waste after food has been digested, removing the rectum made a colostomy necessary. Such waste matter is not poisonous, but room must be made for continuing nourishment. Thus colostomies — surgically created exits for waste — become necessary when the colon is blocked or threatened by blockage (as in colo-rectal cancer). They are also essential when the colon is severely torn or ruptured in an accident or if the colon perforates (tears) as a result of acute *diverticulitis.* A colostomy may also be necessary — usually on a temporary basis — when a child is born without a normal opening at the lower end of the digestive tract (*imperforate anus*).

Any colostomy involves removing (or in some cases disconnecting) part of the colon (large intestine). If the surgery is permanent, rectum and anus are usually also removed.

The lower end of the digestive tract—colon, rectum, and anus — is shaped like a squatty question mark:

This muscular tube, some six feet long, has two main functions. It absorbs a great deal of water (and the minerals dissolved therein) from newly digested food. It also transports and stores residue until a convenient time and place for its disposal. No digestion takes place in the colon.

As food waste enters the colon from the ileum, the last segment of the small intestine, it is generally quite soft, even liquid. However, as this fecal matter makes its clockwise journey up the ascending colon, across the transverse colon, and down the descending and sigmoid colon to the rectum and anus, it becomes firmer as additional water is absorbed.

An individual's colon may be interrupted by a colostomy at any point. Medical reasons for the surgery pinpoint its location; the location is responsible for its name.

How one manages the colostomy depends partly on how liquid or solid the stool is at the chosen site; as little as 8 or 10 inches can make quite a difference in the consistency of the feces. (In spite of appearance, even firmer, "formed" stool is still 3/4 water and 1/4 solid material: undigested roughage, bacteria, some inorganic matter and a little protein. The typical brown color comes from bile.)

No matter where the stoma is located, one thing is missing. The anus, with its ring of muscles which make voluntary control of bowel movements possible, has been either removed or inactivated. With no more voluntary control, the colostomate chooses and learns new techniques of bowel regulation. Regulating the bowels—in a way that's acceptable to the new ostomate—is the secret of living comfortably with a colostomy.

Probably the most difficult kind of ostomy to manage is one located in the transverse colon. Sometimes these are temporary, to allow a section of colon to heal while still permitting regular discharge of feces. Such a colostomy (which can be double-barreled or loop) usually has two stomas next to each other. One discharges feces; the other, still connected to the rectum and anus, secretes some mucus. It often takes months or even longer before damage from a car accident, for instance, has mended, but then the two sections of the colon can be reconnected. Only small scars will mark where the stomas were. In the case of infants, such a temporary colostomy may be used to allow growth before more permanent corrective surgery is done. Sometimes, transverse colostomies are done to make a person more comfortable, even when no cure is possible.

Since this is often emergency surgery, there may not be time for the careful approach of non-emergency ostomies. Stomas are often large, irregular, and hastily constructed; stoma problems occur frequently. The location doesn't help; when the ostomate bends over, appliances are under a great strain. It is difficult to fit an appliance to cover two stomas, and since stool is still quite liquid at this point in its journey, protecting the skin remains essential.

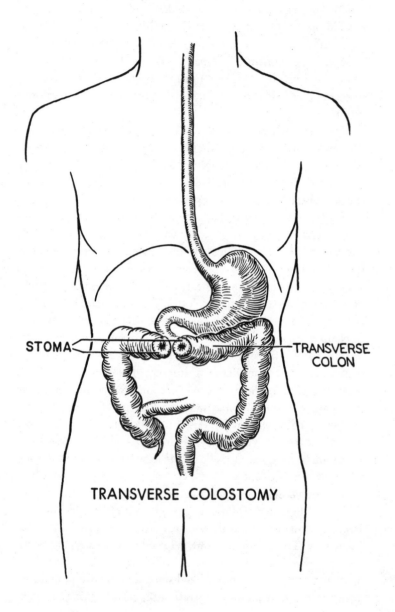

STOMA

TRANSVERSE COLON

TRANSVERSE COLOSTOMY

Sometimes ostomates with a temporary ostomy are inclined to treat it casually, feeling that any skin problems can be solved later, after the colon is reconnected; this can be disastrous.

It's worth a long trip to get an ET's help with these difficult ostomies. The person with a temporary ostomy stays in close contact with the surgeon so that the colon is reconnected as soon as possible.

By far the most common colostomy (and the most common ostomy, for that matter) is the sigmoid colostomy. The principal reason for such surgery is the discovery of a malignancy in the rectum or adjacent colon.

Since the stool at this end of the digestive tract is fairly solid, the sigmoid colostomate has some choices in how to cope with the ostomy: irrigation (basically, an enema through the stoma), diet and exercise, or laissez-faire. For a time, in the United States, there was pressure on all sigmoid colostomates to irrigate. Not to do so was somehow anti-social—almost immoral! But irrigation doesn't work for all sigmoid colostomates (particularly those with an irritable or a very sluggish bowel) and some colostomates just don't like it. Now there's greater emphasis on the colostomate's own choice, based on personal preference, previous patterns of evacuation, and living situation. Many colostomates change or combine methods (switching to laissez-faire and an appliance during a wilderness camping trip, for instance).

With irrigation, the bowel is taught to respond on schedule to the stimulus of water. If this works for a particular ostomate, the unpredictable becomes predictable, and the ostomate can choose the time and place for evacuation. Proper irrigation does *not* wash out the bowel, and has nothing to do with the health of the intestinal tract. What it does is stretch the last section of digestive tract before the stoma; the intestine responds to this stretching by pushing the irrigating fluid out and the indigestible residue with it.

In the United States, irrigation remains a popular method for coping with a sigmoid colostomy (in other countries it is far less

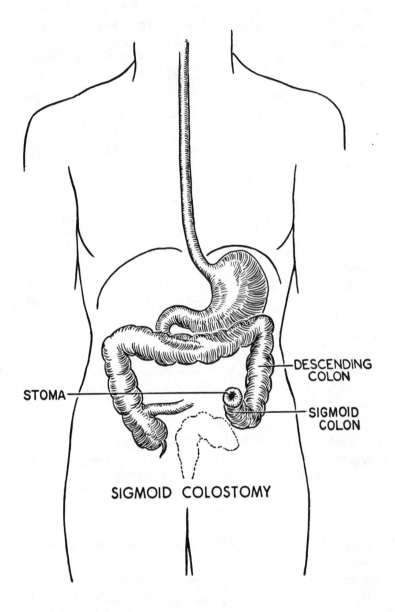

STOMA

DESCENDING
COLON

SIGMOID
COLON

SIGMOID COLOSTOMY

common). If a person prefers irrigation, and the technique works well for him or her, the colostomate can count on regular evacuations, most of the time. Between irrigations, relatively free of the chance of accidents and, thus, of the need for an appliance, the colostomate can wear a small pad, often backed with plastic, to protect the stoma, and to protect clothes from mucus or any discharge. (Some colostomates choose a "security pouch," a small, closed-bottom appliance.) The body feels more like it used to feel. Since the special irrigation equipment lasts for a long time, the expense of appliances is reduced.

A successful irrigation prevents expulsion of feces for at least 24 hours. To achieve this, colostomates irrigate at the same time regularly every day, every other day (or even every third or fourth day), depending on individual bowel pattern.

Instruction from someone who knows how — an ET or a knowledgeable nurse—helps immensely.

Basically, the colostomate uses about a quart of lukewarm water. This runs slowly from a suspended bag through a tube into the stoma. The colostomate hangs the filled bag and tubing from a hook so that the bottom of the bag is at about shoulder height when the colostomate straddles the toilet or sits on a chair facing the toilet. The irrigation process is neat, thanks to an irrigating sleeve which attaches around the stoma. This has an opening near the top for the tube from the suspended bag, and an open end at the bottom to permit discharge of waste into the toilet.

Most colostomates now use a plastic cone on the irrigating tube. This fits snugly into the stoma and prevents any chance of damage to the intestinal lining. The shape of the cone keeps fluid from returning around the cone before the irrigation is completed. Some colostomates still use a catheter tip, lubricate the tip with a non-greasy surgical lubricant—not petroleum jelly—and insert gently with a rolling motion. (The catheter carries more risk of perforating the intestine.) The tubing usually has a clamp to slow or stop the flow of water into the stoma; otherwise, the colostomate can pinch the tubing. Some people experience cramping or nausea during this 5-to-10-minute period of inflow. This should not happen. The usual culprit is too much water, or water that is too cold, or that flows too fast.

After the water finishes flowing in, the colostomate can wait five minutes before gently removing the cone or catheter; the returns come in spurts through the irrigating sleeve into the toilet. This may take 45 minutes or so. After the major portion of the bowel movement returns (usually after 10 or 15 minutes), the colostomate can fold over and clamp the bottom of the irrigating sleeve, and then move around the house, catch up on reading—in short, do whatever passes the time. Before long, the person who irrigates learns how it feels when all the water and bowel movement have been expelled. Then, perhaps, it's time for a bath or shower.

Long sits on a cold toilet seat have brought out the inventor in many a colostomate. Ingenious Ed Gambrell, from Atlanta, put together a board, a four-inch thickness of foam rubber, a sheet of plastic, some tape, and a towel. Adding a terry cloth cover to warm the back of the toilet, he came up with his own "colostothrone," a comfortable skinny seat which fits on the back of the toilet seat. Cutting a U-shaped hole at the front bottom of a large sweat shirt, he had a "colostojacket" to keep him cosy no matter how icy the temperature. Many colostomates use a foot-stool, and now padded toilet seats are sold everywhere. Since relaxation is essential for a successful irrigation, it's worth looking around to see how physical and mental comfort can be increased (radio or TV, or a bookcase, maybe?).

In some households, privacy is a luxury, especially if there are others banging on the bathroom door. If a change in irrigation time doesn't work, the colostomate may decide to compromise. Ed Gambrell insists on privacy when he watches a ball game on TV while he irrigates. Otherwise, he resigns himself to a partial "open door policy." The kids can ask their questions. His cigar smoke can exit. Everyone's happy.

Some bowels never adjust to irrigation. Other people just don't like the whole idea, or prefer to use their time differently. If bowel movements were regular before surgery, the colostomate, with a little judicious attention to diet and exercise, may be able to encourage a tendency toward regularity again. For some people, juggling low residue foods, which tend to be constipating, with high and medium bulk foods can alter the consistency of the discharge, and may make the timing more predictable. This sort of regulation doesn't work at all the first weeks after surgery when there may be almost continual fecal movement. During this early stage, the colostomate wears an appliance all the time. Later, he/she may begin to see a pattern; perhaps more and more and more regularly, the bowel moves after breakfast.

Noting the foods eaten in the previous two or three days, when the bowel moves at an unexpected time, gives the colostomate some idea of what foods to eat or avoid. While some colostomates seem to be able to eat anything, others find they get diarrhea or excessive gas from very spicy foods, foods high in elemental sulphur and iron (onions, cabbage), or other particular kinds of food. (Often people who have trouble with one kind of food at some point can tolerate it later.) Once the colostomy learns to behave docilely, in response to food and exercise, a few colostomates can attach an appliance when the bowel movement is expected, and wear a light covering over the stoma at other times. Most still wear an appliance all the time, however. The records are skimpy, but complete control by diet and exercise appears to be rare. Drugs which slow the bowel are added sometimes, but they have their own hazards. Further experimentation might develop more dependable approaches.

Then there is the laissez-faire approach. This involves wearing an appliance all the time, emptying it when necessary, and otherwise letting the colon go its own way. Some colostomies never respond to irrigation or diet control, and some colostomates just prefer this simple method of management. This method does mean the expense of appliances, however. Since most fecal matter from sigmoid colostomies is fairly solid, and thus doesn't pool on the skin, most colostomates aren't plagued with major skin problems; cleaning gently but thoroughly around the stoma, changing appliances regularly, and keeping away from appliance products which cause allergic skin reactions, help maintain healthy skin around the stoma.

All colostomates may suffer occasionally from *diarrhea* or looseness of stool — from that 24-hour flu bug, an antibiotic, those extra-spicy enchiladas, or as an aftereffect of radiation therapy. Time, a change in diet, and perhaps anti-diarrhea medication usually take care of it. Irrigation should be postponed until the bowel slows down again. This is the time to dig out that emergency drainable appliance.

Constipation (hardness of stool) may be a problem. If the problem continues, the colostomate may want to add more high residue foods to the diet: bran, fruit and vegetables, whole grain breads, for instance. Some of the bulk-producing laxatives can help, as can stool softeners. (The irritating laxatives can cause trouble.) More exercise, a cup of hot liquid, a soothing bath, any relaxing activity, are home remedies for constipation. Pain medications — especially the narcotics — are notorious constipation-causers, as are iron pills. If these are factors, the doctor may be able to suggest a change in medication. In any case, if the problem lasts for a while, it's definitely time to visit the doctor.

For all colostomates, managing this new change in the plumbing is a challenge. Fred E. Bradford, M.D., sums it up: "Learning to manage a colostomy is much simpler than learning to ride a bicycle, and no one ever mastered the bike who quit after the first fall."

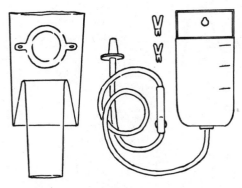

1. An irrigation kit contains a bag for the irrigation water. This bag is attached to a tube which has a clamp to adjust water flow. Many colostomates use a plastic cone at the other end of the tube; this cone fits snugly against the stoma. An irrigating sleeve attaches over the stoma and is long enough to reach into the toilet. Clips allow the colostomate to close the irrigating sleeve after the irrigation process is partially complete.

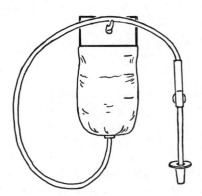

2. With water-flow clamp on the tube closed, the colostomate fills the irrigation bag with a quart or so of lukewarm water and hangs the bag on a sturdy hook; the bottom of the bag will be at shoulder height when the colostomate sits on the toilet or on a chair facing the toilet. The water-flow clamp is released slowly so that water runs through the tube to clear out any air. The clamp is closed again.

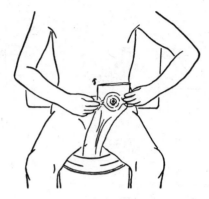

3. The colostomate sits on the toilet or a chair facing the toilet. The irrigating sleeve is placed over the stoma and held in place with a belt. The bottom end of the sleeve rests in the toilet.

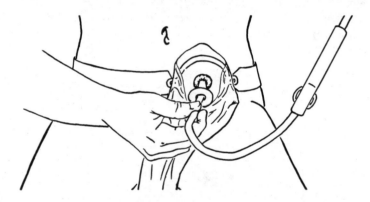

4. The cone is held in place firmly against the stoma. If the colostomate uses an irrigating tip instead of the cone, the distance the tip is to be inserted into the ostomy is measured and marked on the tube beforehand; the tip is then covered with a non-greasy surgical lubricant and inserted into the stoma with a gentle, rolling motion. A *dam* (a flat, doughnut-shaped device that encircles the irrigating tube) is held against the stoma to keep water from escaping around the sides of the irrigation tip.

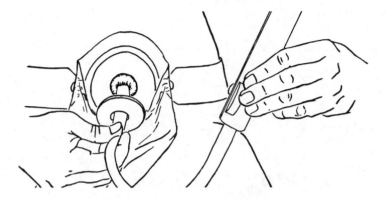

5. The water-flow clamp is opened slowly to allow a gentle stream of water to enter the stoma; it takes five to ten minutes for all the water to flow in. The colostomate then waits five or so more minutes before removing the cone or irrigating tip; this extra wait gives a more complete irrigation.

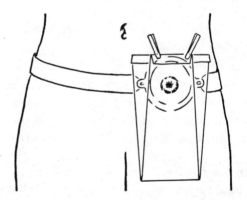

6. The cone or irrigating tip is removed from the ostomy. Most of the irrigation returns come in spurts into the toilet during the first few minutes. After this period, the colostomate can close the open ends of the irrigating sleeve and can attend to other business. When the irrigation is complete, the irrigating sleeve is removed, a soft pad or security pouch is applied over the stoma, and the irrigation equipment is cleaned.

CHAPTER 10 Ileostomies: Living with an Almost Instant Cure

So much of my life had been devoted to an ulcerated colon which no longer exists . . . such a waste of time.
Norbert Hertel, ileostomate

If you ever need to find the nearest bathroom in a strange town, seek out the person with chronic inflammatory bowel disease. Along with his mental map of every bathroom in town, he can probably tell you about the local hospitals: he's been in them enough.

But, no matter how much the disease has disrupted his life, when the typical person with inflammatory bowel disease hears about the hope an ileostomy may offer, he balks. So may his family and even his doctor. If it becomes a life-or-death choice, he still despairs: "An ostomy? How can I live with something. . . like that?"

After surgery and recovery, he asks a different question: "Why did I *ever* wait so long?"

Although there's no such thing as a *typical* ostomate, those who have had ileostomies share some striking similarities. Most are young and undergo surgery after devastating sieges of inflammatory bowel disease. And most, after recovering from surgery, resume life—whether school, career, raising a family or whatever—with abundant energy and enthusiasm.

Such happy endings are relatively new.

Inflammatory bowel diseases have been around for a long time. Bonnie Prince Charlie supposedly suffered from one, as did Beethoven. Roman Emperor Claudius had the symptoms of "the bloody flux" and, as Dr. F. T. de Domnal reports, a physician from Ephesus (namely, incredibly, *Soranus!*) wrote a quite adequate description of the disease in 117 A.D.

Inflammatory bowel disease is a catch-all phrase for several diseases which attack the intestinal tract. If the colon (large intestine) is the target organ, the disease is called *colitis.* Ulcerative colitis, the most common chronic form of colitis, usually starts in the rectum and spreads upward, battering the inner lining of the large intestine. Unpredictably, the disease flares and recedes, destroying the mucous lining of the large intestine in bouts of severe, often bloody, diarrhea.

The deeper layers of the bowel are attacked in *Crohn's disease,* also commonly called *ileitis* (when it involves mostly the ileum, the lower half of the small intestine), or *regional enteritis* (from the Greek word, *enteron,* meaning "intestine"), or *granulomatous disease of the bowel* (from the appearance of the diseased intestine under a microscope).

Doctors diagnose about 100,000 new cases of inflammatory bowel disease each year—and perhaps another 100,000 milder cases go undiagnosed. Most victims of inflammatory bowel disease are young, and many have a relative with the disease. These diseases sometimes attack other parts of the body, too, including joints, liver, and eyes, although the intestine takes the brunt of the assault. The risk of bowel cancer rises for people who have had long-term ulcerative colitis.

No one is sure yet just why someone gets inflammatory bowel disease. In 1966, the National Foundation of Ileitis & Colitis, Inc.

was formed to help find out why. The Foundation raises money for research into causes and treatment.

At the moment, the most popular theory is that the body, for some reason, begins to see the bowel as foreign, as not belonging to itself. The body then does everything in its power to get rid of this "enemy" bowel. But why does the body suddenly reject the bowel? Some researchers are looking at the possibility of a slow reaction to a virus or bacteria (perhaps the dog distemper virus in Crohn's disease), or to some toxin. Emotional factors may play a role, but few researchers feel they are the *cause* of the disease.

Perhaps, in their research into these and similar "auto-immune" diseases (like rheumatoid arthritis), in which the body attacks part of itself, scientists will find some way to persuade the body to recognize the bowel again as part of itself. Until that day, doctors give supportive care, prescribing anti-diarrhea drugs and pain medications, for instance, or replacing fluids during an acute attack. They may use *corticosteroids*, very powerful drugs which don't cure the disease but may ease some of the symptoms.

For most patients, this supportive treatment works well. But for those with more severe disease, who need heavy, constant doses of drugs, the treatment becomes almost as bad as the disease. As artist Reba Dockterman recalls about the years before her ileostomy: "There was little dignity left in my life as poverty took over, only over-shadowed by pain.

"The years inched by. I was no longer a model, a job I'd enjoyed with pride before my illness gave me a bloated tummy and my drugs puffed my cheeks into a moon-shaped face. My skin was modulated between shades of red to violet, my fingernails were completely concave, and the dark circles under my eyes could not be covered by the heaviest of makeups."

Reba brought up the possibility of ostomy surgery to her doctor. Like many doctors, he hesitated, because, "I'd hate to do that to you unless I have to." Finally, however, after the many hospitalizations, weight loss, dehydration, constant pain, weakening, utter misery, bleeding, harrowing social consequences

—all common experiences for those with severe inflammatory bowel disease—Reba had an ileostomy.

Until the last few years, she wouldn't have had that option. In the 1890's, two English doctors reported separately on two surgeries for cancer that may have been ileostomies. In 1913, Dr. John Young Brown in St. Louis constructed the first ileostomy in the U.S. At that point, and for many years to come, an ileostomy remained a real horror story. Patients became dehydrated and died. With a primitive arsenal of medicines, surgeons watched their patients die of infection. Those who survived had towels and pads and whatever they could improvise to contain drainage. One company made "appliances"—bulky, rubber, poorly-fitted pouches.

Gradually the picture brightened. British surgeon Bryan Brooke devised the Brooke ileostomy in the early 1950's: no longer was ileostomy surgery "a living death." Surgeon Rupert Turnbull, of the Cleveland Clinic, brought the Brooke procedure to the United States. Medical advances such as antibiotics helped. Surgery could provide at last an almost instant cure for intolerable disease.

An ileostomy is an artificial opening on the abdominal wall through which body wastes can be expelled. A surgeon removes or disconnects the diseased colon (and in some cases of Crohn's disease, perhaps also a hefty section of the small intestine) and brings the end of the ileum (the last portion of the small intestine) through the abdominal wall to form a stoma, usually on the lower right side of the abdomen. During the same surgery, or later, the rectum and anus may also be removed; in any case, they no longer function. (If they are left in, rectum and anus are checked periodically by the doctor; in ulcerative colitis, they may become diseased after several years.) An external appliance substitutes for the old storage area of colon and rectum.

Since 1969, Swedish surgeon Nils Kock has been experimenting with a continent ileostomy, a "Kock pouch," with which the ileostomate does not need to wear an appliance. In this surgery, which usually isn't done for patients with Crohn's disease

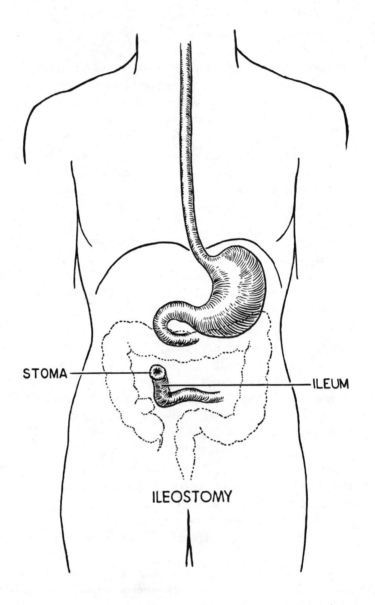

STOMA

ILEUM

ILEOSTOMY

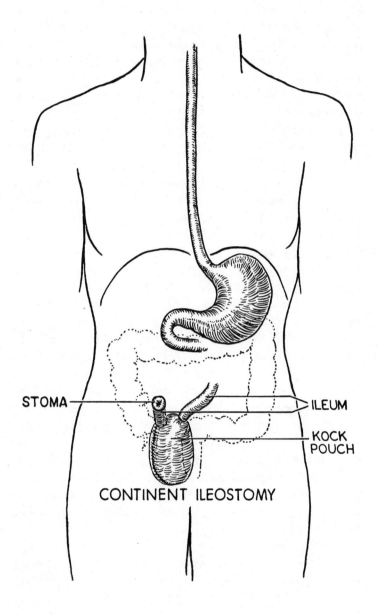

STOMA

ILEUM

KOCK
POUCH

CONTINENT ILEOSTOMY

and to date is suitable only for certain people, the surgeon loops part of the ileum back on itself and constructs from this loop a reservoir pouch *inside* the abdomen. Then the doctor builds a one-way valve from the reservoir to the abdominal wall, through which the ileostomate inserts a catheter a few times a day to drain the reservoir. The reservoir stretches gradually until it holds a pint or more.

Whether a person undergoes ileostomy surgery for inflammatory bowel disease or for less common problems like birth defects of bowel or anus, *familial polyposis* (an inherited disease in which the bowel becomes cancerous if not removed during young adulthood), injury or cancer, he needs plenty of physical help and emotional support. Inflammatory bowel disease patients probably need some building up before surgery, perhaps through intravenous feeding (including *total parenteral nutrition*, in which proteins, carbohydrates, vitamins and minerals and sometimes fats are given through a large blood vessel). Medicine may need to be changed, especially if the patient has been taking high doses of steroids, which would slow wound healing.

In retrospect, those first few days after an ileostomy seem unreal. Jane Walker, an ET from Atlanta, Georgia, writes: "It is difficult, many times, for us to remember what it is like to be a new ileostomate. Looking back, do you remember the first feelings of something 'alive' on your abdomen as you experienced the peristaltic action of the stoma? How about the feeling of warm stool draining into the disposable pouch, wondering if it was 'in or out' of the pouch and looking to see? Did you carry a sack full of supplies everywhere you went, afraid you would break a seal? Do you remember, in your early post-op days, holding your hand on your pouch or stoma when you walked. Don't kid yourself, you did too, and probably still do at times."

But those first days pass quickly. One day the new ileostomate realizes he or she has gone *thirty minutes* without even being aware of the ostomy! Confidence builds. The ostomate masters techniques for emptying and changing appliances, or for draining the Kock pouch if he has a continent ileostomy. Before long, such chores are just part of the daily routine, along with brushing one's teeth.

Ileostomates share some concerns of colostomates — like odor (see Chapter 12: "Appliances") and gas (Chapter 13: "Eating Well"). And, like those colostomates with ostomies not far from the ileum who also have a relatively liquid stool, ileostomates have to keep an eye on replenishing water and salt. Also, food blockage of the intestine and, for those who have had a large portion of the small intestine removed, vitamin B-12 absorption may become problems (Chapter 13: "Eating Well"). Like colostomates, ileostomates who have had rectum and anus removed have a perineal wound which may be tender for a time (Chapter 6: "On the Mend").

But ileostomates have some special challenges, mostly from the nature of body waste when it reaches the stoma.

The body functions quite nicely without the colon and rectum, but it has lost some of its ability to absorb water. Waste will still be quite liquid when it reaches the stoma; eventually the ileum learns to take over most of the water-absorbing function of the colon, and the stool will become thicker, perhaps pasty in consistency. The kidneys continue to adjust the water balance and the urine may become more concentrated as the body loses water in the stool. Drinking *lots* of fluids does *not* make the feces more liquid, and *does* help the kidneys wash out the chemicals which can lead to kidney stones, a hazard for long-term ileostomates.

Until the digestive tract starts functioning again after surgery (usually a few days), there's no stool. When *peristalsis* (the muscular contractions which move food and waste matter through the digestive system) finally returns, the ostomy is often on its *worst* behavior. Stool may be constant and watery.

Time tames many ileostomies. But it's an individual matter. Some ileostomates can set a clock by their stomas: half an hour after they eat, "Vesuvius" erupts. Others, including many of those who have had some of the small intestine removed at the same time, continue to have more constant or unpredictable discharge. For many, there are predictable times of peace, especially during the later morning hours.

The small intestine's specialty is digesting food, breaking it up into tiny pieces with the help of enzymes. Given a chance, those same intestinal enzymes which will digest a New York steak will do the same thing to any skin they touch.

When fashioning the ostomy, the surgeon ideally creates a stoma which extends 3/4 to one inch beyond the abdomen. Thus, the ileum discharges directly into the appliance and away from the skin. But the ileostomate takes special care to protect the skin around the stoma and to keep the appliance seal secure. Cleaning the area well but gently, using adhesives or skin barriers to which the skin is tolerant, watching for any break in the seal which means an appliance change is necessary—all these contribute to healthy skin.

Time-release and other coated medicine capsules and pills, and some other kinds of tablets which are absorbed in the colon, may pass whole through the ileostomate's system. Many medicines are available in liquid form; some others can be removed from capsules. The doctor or pharmacist can advise. The ostomate should remind the doctor or pharmacist to provide medication in the right form.

Mae West said it: "When choosing between two evils, I always like to try the one I've never tried before."

An ileostomy's no evil—as thousands of ileostomates can attest —although it's certainly new and strange and unfamiliar at first. But when one remembers what the ileostomy replaces. . . .

As Michele says, "Anyone who wants the battered, tortured intestine I got rid of, is more than welcome to it! I don't hurt any more. I can eat. I can work. Sure, sometimes it's a bother—but I love my ileostomy.

"I can *live* now!"

CHAPTER 11 ❄ *Life Without a*
Built-in Bladder

The urinary stoma is the only stoma that is connected directly to
a life supporting system — the kidneys.
Katherine F. Jeter, ET

People who have a urostomy — a surgical opening in the
abdominal wall so that urine is diverted away from a diseased or
defective part of the urinary tract—come in all different sizes and
ages. Baby Steve, cooing and drooling like any five-month-old, is
a veteran urostomate already because he was born without a
bladder. Six-year-old Patti Anne treasures her new ruffled panties
— a urostomy spells freedom from constant diapers and "Baby,
Baby, Patti!" taunts from her playmates; a spinal defect meant
that she couldn't control urination before her surgery. Jim, 22,
needs a temporary urostomy until he grows strong enough to
withstand major repair of car accident injuries to his urinary tract.
To 55-year-old Tom, a urostomy means he has exchanged a
cancerous bladder for an external appliance, and a new lease on
life.

Whatever the difference in their immediate reasons for surgery,
Steve, Patti Anne, Jim and Tom (and thousands of others like

them) all became urostomates to provide a safe and reliable passageway out of the body for urine.

Twenty-four hours a day, a veritable Niagara of blood rushes through the two kidneys, small but essential organs, one on each side of the spinal column. Each minute, an adult male's kidneys filter about five cups of blood through two million nephrons, tiny processing stations which flush waste, and then return the purified blood to the circulatory system. Responding to hormones, the kidneys also maintain the balance of water and other substances like sodium and potassium in the body.

Each kidney empties urine it has made into a ureter, a narrow, muscular tube which propels the fluid, with a milking action, through a special one-way valve into the bladder. The bladder is basically a reservoir, supplied with muscle and nerves, to hold urine until it is convenient to dispose of it. From the bladder, urine travels through the urethra, a simple passageway to the outside. The nerve supply to the urethra makes it open and close at the right times.

This whole system is a sterile one; urine leaving the body should be completely free of bacteria. Even if infection reaches the bladder through the urethra, ordinarily the one-way valve on each ureter protects the kidneys.

At least some kidney function, and some means of removing the urine from the body, are essential for life. Any condition which seriously interrupts the flow of urine to the outside can lead to an ostomy. Where in the urinary tract, and how the surgery is done give the particular ostomy its name.

Some surgeries are relatively easy and straightforward, and are now performed primarily on patients who are quite weak and ill. In a *nephrostomy* (from the Greek for "kidney"), a tube is inserted directly into the kidney to bring urine to the outside. A *ureterostomy* means that the ureter is brought through the abdominal wall. In a *vesicostomy* or *cystostomy* (both terms come from ancient words for "bladder"), the bladder opens quite directly on the abdominal wall.

Relatively simple operations these may be, but they present so many difficulties after surgery that they are rare except for emergencies. When it is brought to the surface of the body, the narrow ureter tends to scar and close off. The vesicostomy, because of its location in the pubic area, becomes quite difficult to manage; pubic hair and shape of the lower pelvis make appliances hard to attach and maintain. And the closer the ostomy is to the kidney, the smaller is the margin of safety for protecting the kidney from infection.

People who require a urinary ostomy and can tolerate more complicated surgery need something more. In the early 20th century, surgeons began experimenting with using a portion of the intestine to form a conduit, or passageway, to the outside. In early attempts, urine was diverted into the sigmoid colon where the anal sphincter could provide control. Dr. Arthur I. Murphy, of Pittsburg, claims: "It has been said that patients with this procedure — *ureterosigmoidostomy* — were sick twice a year, six months at a time." Miraculously, however, especially in a time before antibiotics, a few people actually survived and thrived; how they avoided the profound changes in body chemistry and the kidney infections from bacteria in the colon which killed others, remains a mystery.

Dr. Bricker gets credit for developing, in the 1940s and 50s, what remains the most common urinary diversion — the *ileal conduit* (also known as "Bricker's pouch"). Although the surgery is complicated, the idea is simple. A 6-8–inch piece near the end of the *ileum* (the last part of the small intestine) is isolated, together with its blood supply. The rest of the small intestine is reconnected, so that bowel movements pass normally. The segment of the ileum can then be moved, along with its nerve and blood supply, so that ureters can be attached to it; the surgeon sews shut one end of the segment and fashions the other into a stoma on the abdominal wall.

Depending on the condition for which surgery is done and the particular procedure, the surgeon may or may not remove the

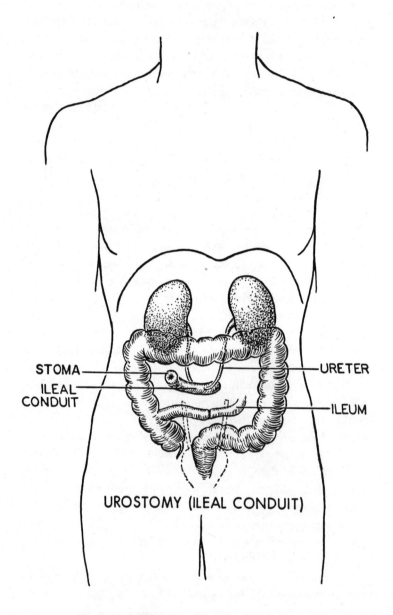

STOMA

ILEAL
CONDUIT

URETER

ILEUM

UROSTOMY (ILEAL CONDUIT)

bladder. The detached segment of ileum serves as a passageway for urine to the outside. Since the blood supply remains, the segment continues peristalsis, the normal intestinal pulsation to keep the urine moving away from the kidneys. Since an ileal conduit is *not* an artificial bladder, one needs an appliance, securely fastened to the skin, to act as a bladder; the emptying spout of the appliance takes the place of the urethra. The normal kidney produces an average of 10-15 drops of urine each minute around the clock, so drainage is constant.

The ileal conduit is still far from a perfect solution (although it works remarkably well). The one-way valve from ureter to bladder is missing, so the kidneys have limited protection from urine backflow and possible infection.

Surgeons continue to modify the ileal conduit and to explore new ways of getting urine from inside to outside with minimal bother. Using others parts of the intestine, like a segment of colon —the so-called *colonic conduit*—is becoming more popular. Some surgeons are experimenting with using several layers of the muscular colon to form a one-way valve to keep urine from backing up into the ureters from the conduit. An internal pouch from which urine could be drained periodically with a catheter is another area for exploration. For those with damage to the nerves which control urination, a bladder pacemaker (an electronic device which signals when the bladder needs emptying), is yet another possibility.

Those first days after surgery can be a bit harrowing. The appliance, frequently from a limited hospital stock, may be cumbersome or ill-fitting. It will be hooked up to a bedside receptacle all the time at first. Eventually, the new urostomate learns to empty the appliance regularly; then it is connected to the bedside receptacle only at night. Eventually, too, he/she gets a good, comfortable, workable appliance, though that may take some trial and error.

New urostomates, deluged with a mass of information, may find that separating the crucial from the less important seems overwhelming at first, but it is not as complicated as it appears.

The *most* important consideration for any urostomate is to keep those kidneys functioning smoothly; this must be a real *commitment*. In most urostomies done currently, the kidneys empty, after a brief passage with no one-way valves, into an outside appliance. This means less protection from infection, more chance of urine backing up into the kidneys with a load of bacteria. Fortunately, in most cases, with good care, no problem develops.

But preventing kidney infection involves some common-sense measures. If the urine flows well, and stays away from the stoma, infection is rare. This means checking fairly often that urine continues to flow. One hour without urine is too long for a urostomate—medical help is necessary. Bacteria multiply rapidly in urine. This means using *clean* appliances, either disposables or reusables, thoroughly scrubbed and soaked in the solution suggested by the manufacturer, or in equal parts of white vinegar and tap water for twenty minutes or so, then rinsed completely and dried. Meticulous care of appliances is an absolute necessity for the person with a urostomy. Emptying appliances frequently makes sense too, so that old urine never comes in contact with the opening of the stoma.

During the day when people stand or sit, gravity draws urine away from the stoma. During sleep, or other long bed rest, urostomates connect the bottom of the appliance to tubing which attaches in turn to some kind of bedside receptacle, perhaps a large vinyl bag made for that purpose which hooks over the bed frame, or a half gallon jug modified and placed on the floor inside a wastebasket or other covering. Gravity continues to keep urine away from the stoma so that infection can't get a toehold.

To avoid creating a vacuum in the system, a small amount of fluid is left in the appliance before connecting to the night drainage. Also, urostomates secure the tubing at the top of the vented bottle so that no more than one inch of it extends into the bottle; should the level of urine rise above the bottom of the tubing, drainage stops.

Urostomates have a few strategies for keeping infection at bay. They know that bacteria thrive in concentrated, alkaline urine— so they turn the tables. They drink *lots* of fluids (good advice for most people), at least eight or ten glasses a day. They never pass a drinking fountain without stopping! This keeps the urine dilute, and flowing swiftly away from the kidneys.

Too, people with urostomies are urged to work at keeping their urine on the acid side, and hence unfriendly to bacteria. A glass or two of cranberry juice or a bowl of cranberry sauce each day does this nicely; Vitamin C tablets may be prescribed by the doctor for the same purpose. (Surprisingly enough, orange juice or other citrus *doesn't work*. since it becomes alkaline in the body).

Dipping a special test paper into urine tests how acid or alkaline the urine is; this is called the pH of the urine, and the doctor or other health professional can give directions for using it, if advisable. To be an accurate test, the urine must be fresh and not on the stoma (which is alkaline). A good time to check is during an appliance change when a drop of urine drains from the stoma.

Urostomates should learn the signs and symptoms of possible urinary tract infection and report for medical care *immediately* if any of these occur: fever, chills, flank or abdominal pain, bloody or tea-colored urine, foul smelling or "thick" whitish urine. (People with an ileal or a colonic conduit will normally have threads of mucus in the urine, since the intestinal segment continues to secrete mucus; this should not be confused with pus and infection.)

Regular check-ups include urinalysis and a blood test to see that the kidneys are functioning well. Doctors schedule periodic IVPs (intravenous pyelogram—a kidney and urinary tract x-ray) if the urostomate tolerates them; otherwise different tests are used. It's a good idea for the ostomate to plan a long-term check-up schedule with the doctor.

No matter how complicated this all seems at first, it soon becomes as much second nature as brushing and flossing teeth. And, in fact, keeping urine flowing well, and away from the stoma, means no problem with infection for most urostomates.

The other fundamental concern for urostomates is the nature of urine and its flow. Urine flows everywhere. It wanders into the tiniest holes in the appliance seal. Urine on uncovered skin causes few problems, but urine on skin *under* any appliance seal causes many problems.

Expert instruction on applying the pouch, appropriate skin preparations and/or skin barriers, and a properly fitted appliance (followed by supervised practice, and then reasonable care in applying pouches) forestalls most difficulties. Preventing irritation or healing it at the first hint of trouble is important.

Urine that is alkaline fosters infection; it also causes crystals to encrust on and around the stoma. These are scratchy and irritating. Using the proper opening diameter on the appliance and acidifying the urine cure this. In the meantime, putting two ounces of vinegar-water solution (½ cup white vinegar to 1 quart water) through the outlet valve of the emptied appliance, with an infant ear syringe or similar device, twice a day, and lying down for 20 minutes allows the solution to dissolve the crystals on the stoma.

Urine contains dissolved minerals and some other substances which tend to form stones in some people. Drinking abundant fluids, and, if the doctor recommends it, cutting down on certain foods, may solve this problem. (Which food to restrict depends on which minerals cause problems in a particular individual.)

The final concern of urine flow is that it's constant. At first this may make keeping a dry stoma area while changing an appliance seem impossible, but urostomates quickly discover such useful devices as a tampon, or pill bottle of proper size filled with cotton, to cover the stoma during changes. Most urostomates change appliances every five to seven days, but that's an individual matter. (Many could go longer, but it's important to change to a clean appliance at least once a week.)

(Sometimes doctors, and others, call an "ileal conduit" an "ileostomy" — which confuses everyone. Basically, if an ostomy which involves the ileum produces urine, it's an ileal conduit; if it produces feces, it's an ileostomy.)

Since a urostomy is connected directly to organs essential for life, proper care is even more urgent than it is with other ostomies. But, that commitment made, the urostomate can start *living* with a urostomy: working, playing, loving. No longer a urostomy which just happens to have a person attached, he can become a *person* who just happens to have a urostomy.

CHAPTER 12 ❖ *Appliances and the Skin They Touch*

Understanding human needs is half the job of meeting them.
Adlai Stevenson

Not many years ago, a lady made her first visit to a stoma clinic —to ask where she could buy good rubber gloves, like "the kind they used to make." Twenty-five years ago, when she had had her surgery, her nurse had suggested taping a rubber glove over the new stoma to collect the body waste. The woman had been doing it ever since, but she couldn't find any good rubber gloves anymore. She wept when she found out how many easier and better ways there are now.

Another ostomate startled his new doctor by displaying the collection device he'd developed and worn for some time: a cigar box, carefully waterproofed. There are several stories of ostomates using a hot water bottle, slit to cover the stoma.

And only a few years ago, according to a story we were told, a delegate from India came to a UOA conference and was proud because he'd learned to cope with his ostomy — by taping an empty tuna fish can on his belly.

That a delegate could travel from India to the United States wearing a tuna fish can says something rather remarkable about human spirit and ingenuity. But it's infinitely easier to manage with a secure, comfortable, and inconspicuous appliance, an ostomate's passport back to the normal world.

For anyone with a stoma, an appliance is a device designed to collect body waste as it's discharged, and to hold it until a convenient time for disposal. Although there are many variations, an ostomy appliance is basically a thin-walled pouch that, when not in use, looks like an off-duty balloon. It is adhered to the skin, sometimes with a separate faceplate (a piece of plastic, rubber, metal, or other material, that resembles a flattened doughnut, with a hole in the center slightly larger than the stoma).

Ostomy appliances aren't new. Probably the first colostomy pouch was a small leather bag designed in 1795 by a French surgeon, Daguesceau, for a patient on whom he had performed sigmoid colon surgery.

But until the late 1940's, with the coming of antibiotics, most surgeons shied away from ostomy surgery. The few patients who survived relied on bulky pads and dressings. One company supplied a cumbersome rubber appliance during the early 1900's.

The choice between smelly piles of dressings and heavy rubber appliances wasn't enough for the ever-increasing group of ostomates in the late 1940's and after. Now that surgeons were doing more surgeries, and many more patients were surviving and expecting to resume a reasonably normal life, ostomates began demanding lightweight, odor-resistant, secure coverings. Plastics entered the scene at about the same time.

Several old-line hospital supply companies began to develop special products for ostomates, and discovered they had stumbled onto a growth industry. Other ostomy appliances and supplies were developed and marketed by ostomates who were frustrated in their own searches for something that really worked.

The ostomate, once stymied by the lack of choices, may be bewildered now by the huge variety of appliances available:

reusable, disposable, one-piece, two-piece, transparent, opaque, plain, fancy. The mind reels!

The goal is an appliance which fits properly, is comfortable, adheres well, is odor proof, non-irritating to the skin, secure, and collects the output until a convenient time for emptying. It's a big order, but more and more people are finding the right appliance for themselves.

Some old-timers stick to an old favorite. Carol, for instance, really feels most comfortable with her sturdy black rubber, gas-valve appliance. Other ostomates want to try everything. One ET, himself an ostomate, is working his way through all the ileostomy appliances and combinations of equipment available, so that he can advise his clients better and increase his own comfort.

Basically, the kind of appliance depends on the kind of surgery, and the kind of person who has the ostomy. If the person has had a urostomy, for instance, he or she needs an appliance to catch and

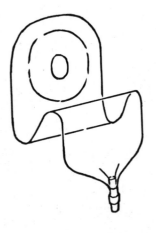

Urostomy appliance collects urine; water-tight valve at bottom is drained frequently.

hold a constant discharge of urine, and to protect the skin around the stoma from urine. A valve at the bottom of the pouch keeps urine in the appliance and releases it easily when the valve is opened for emptying. Special water-resistant adhesives hold the appliance securely around the stoma.

Ileostomates, with a liquid or semi-solid waste usually discharged at frequent times during the day, also need an appliance which can be emptied easily. (Non-stick spray or a drop of baby oil, placed in the bottom of a pouch after emptying and spread along the lower sides, makes it easier to empty later.) The drainage opening must be larger than those made for urostomies.

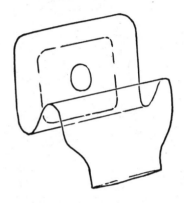

The ileostomy appliance collects stool; some kind of device at the bottom may be opened easily, closed securely. Bottom opening must be large enough so feces can pass through it. Some colostomates wear a similar appliance if stool is loose enough or if colostomate prefers a drainable pouch.

Here the danger to the skin around the stoma comes from enzymes in the stool. Whatever holds the appliance to the skin need not be waterproof, but must protect the skin from enzyme damage.

Colostomates with ostomies in the ascending or transverse colon usually have liquid or semi-solid stools; they need the same kind of appliance as the ileostomate. Also, no matter where in the colon the surgery is, most *new* colostomates have unpredictable stools.

But the colostomate with surgery in the descending or sigmoid colon eventually may have a stool much like the one before surgery. If he or she irrigates, and has little or no discharge between irrigations, a soft square absorbent material, perhaps with a plastic backing, can be used. For more security, many colostomates choose a small disposable closed appliance, which is changed when necessary, usually daily. Skin protection is less of a

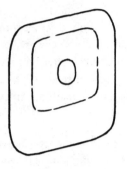

A security pouch for a colostomy collects any drainage between irrigations. It cannot be emptied but is small and compact.

problem for most colostomates since the stool is more solid and thus less likely to pool on the skin. In case of a bout of diarrhea, however, the skin is definitely in danger.

In fact, however, skin care is a major concern for *all* ostomates. As Katherine Jeter, ET, says: "The stoma will take care of itself; you must take care of your skin."

Dr. Logan Clendening ventured close to poetry when he described the skin, one of the most complex organs in the body. Skin, he said, is "... one of the most interesting and mystic structures ... that outer rampart which separates us from the rest of the universe, the sack which contains that juice or essence which is me, or which is you, a moat defensive against insects, poisons, germs ... The very storms of the soul are recorded on it."

The skin around the stoma (peristomal skin) is subject to new substances and stresses after surgery. Irritating discharge from an ostomy (digestive enzymes, for instance, or urine from a urostomy) can devastate any skin it touches.

When one closes off the skin under an appliance to air—even with new porous appliance materials that "breathe" — perspiration may irritate the skin. The warm, moist environment both in and underneath an appliance encourages bacteria and fungi to thrive; if they can reach a raw area on the skin under an appliance, they'll seize the opportunity.

Why is it so important to keep the skin in top condition? Comfort for one reason. Irritated, weepy skin *hurts.* Security is another motive. Sound, smooth skin provides the ideal surface for an appliance, which may adhere poorly to rough, injured skin. Odor builds up also, when bacteria or other particles linger on irritated skin. Health is yet another factor; neither infected skin nor broken skin (which lets the wrong substances into and out of the body) is good for anyone.

Victor Alter, RN, ET, says "Your skin should be absolutely healthy underneath that pouch and should look just the same as it does anywhere else. Not like a football, not like a raw tomato, not like eggplant—nothing—just good healthy skin."

Prevention is the best method for keeping the skin healthy.

There are three layers of skin. The outer layer (or *epidermis*) is made up of dry, dead cells, which are constantly being shed, and the layer of new cells which are growing to replace them. Since serious skin problems usually involve the layers under the epidermis, the trick for the ostomate is to protect the epidermis.

Cleanliness is the foundation of a skin care program, and water is the simplest and safest of all cleaners. Even the mildest soap can add problems unless every bit of it is rinsed away after use.

Scheduling an appliance change at bath or shower time gives the peristomal skin a chance to air and to be washed, gently and

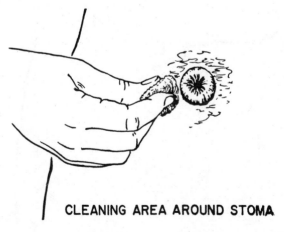

CLEANING AREA AROUND STOMA

thoroughly. This helps keep odor at bay, and washes away some problem-causers, including bacteria and irritating urine crystals (in a urostomy) or digestive enzymes (in an ileostomy). After washing, the skin is patted dry, not rubbed.

Approaching the skin gently is the second step in a sensible skin care program. If an appliance begins to leak, it must be changed (patching doesn't work, since irritating enzymes or urine remain under the appliance seal to damage skin). On the other hand, too-frequent changes don't help, and ripping an appliance off roughly definitely injures the skin. Especially if worn frequently, a tight belt on an appliance can "shear," or pull away, the top layer of the skin from the next layer.

Many ostomates protect the delicate skin around the stoma with a skin barrier.

Several years ago, Dr. Rupert Turnbull of the Cleveland Clinic accidentally spilled a container of *karaya* denture powder on himself. As he tried to clean his hands, he discovered that the karaya became a kind of mucilage as it became wet. Serendipity! Karaya, made from the sap of a species of tree from India, became the great granddaddy of skin barriers for ostomates. Still used widely as powder, paste or solid sheet, it expands as heat from the

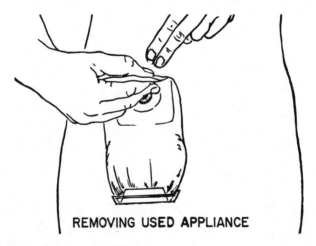

REMOVING USED APPLIANCE

body hits it and molds it to the body surface, protecting the skin from enzymes or other harmful irritants. It gives off acetic acid as it "melts," discouraging bacteria or fungus infection.

Manufacturers have modified karaya by adding other ingredients to it. Or they have used different ingredients entirely to produce other skin barriers which protect the skin and keep the appliance securely in place.

Finding the right skin barrier involves some trial and error. An ET is the best resource for finding out, for instance, which ones are water-soluble and won't work for urostomates, or which ones cause fewest skin senstivities. New products appear constantly, including protective sprays and gels, and it may take experimentation to find the right product, particularly for those with sensitive skin or allergies.

A patch test is the safest way to experiment first. This involves applying a small quantity of the substance in question to the skin on the abdomen away from the stoma, taping it in place, and leaving it for 48 hours. If there is any redness, burning, itching, or other discomfort, the skin is sensitive to the item; if there is no irritation, the product should be safe to use near the stoma. Allergy may develop after the long use of a product. But what appears to be an allergic reaction is often irritation from the product rubbing against the skin.

The next step in a skin care program is getting an appliance which fits. ET Katherine Jeter claims that 99% of skin problems can be avoided if one wears a correctly fitted appliance.

The right size opening for the ring or faceplate around the stoma is crucial. The diameter, or measurement across the largest part of the opening, should be 1/16th to 1/8th of an inch larger than the diameter of the stoma (colostomates with a solid stool don't have to be quite so precise); this gives the stoma a little elbow room to expand when it's discharging waste. Appliance companies supply cards with cut-out rings to measure the stoma. The smallest size which fits without touching the stoma is the right size. Many people with ostomies order appliances by stoma size,

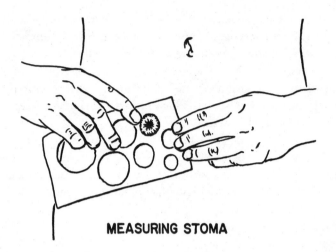

MEASURING STOMA

after measuring with the cut-out rings (a 1¼-inch appliance, for example). Some of those with less regularly-shaped stomas buy appliances and cut out the opening themselves, using a pattern.

However it is achieved, the right size opening in the faceplate means the stoma itself is not irritated by rubbing, and there is just a tiny ring of unprotected skin around the stoma. That tiny margin of skin, along with the skin under the faceplate of the appliance, can then be protected with one of the skin barriers; these are designed to cover *all* the skin around the stoma, leaving absolutely no skin unprotected.

If the skin rebels, even after all this tender loving care, what then? Enzymes, heat, urine, bacteria, and fungi all cause different problems. Sometimes extra care in drying slightly reddened skin (perhaps with the "air" setting of a portable hair dryer) may be enough, or a fresh appliance may work. In most cases, the faster the ostomate seeks the help of an ET or a doctor, the better.

Weepy or broken skin around a stoma is beyond the scope of home remedies. Unless they're cared for immediately, skin problems tend to get worse, in a vicious cycle: the appliance adheres less well to the roughened skin, allowing more enzymes or

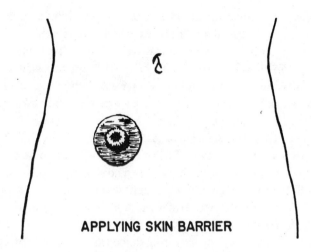

APPLYING SKIN BARRIER

urine to reach the skin, which becomes still more irritated, which then. . . .

Fitting an appliance correctly, essential as it is, presents challenges. If the stoma does not protrude too far and is regularly shaped on a reasonably flat surface, away from prominent bones or scars, on a fairly slender abdomen, a standard appliance should fit well. Otherwise, with help from an ET or other knowledgeable person, the ostomate learns to build up a flat area around the stoma, using pieces of assorted materials like karaya. An oval rather than round faceplate can compensate for a stoma placed too close to a bone or scar. A convex faceplate can help with a too-short or flush stoma.

Not only the anatomy of a particular patient, but financial status, sharpness of vision, overall energy and mobility, and life style are among the important factors for the ostomate choosing an appliance. The athlete, the young child who seems to outgrow appliances faster than T-shirts—in fact everyone, for some reason or other, has special needs in choosing an appliance.

There are many ways to get a bird's eye view of what is available. Most UOA chapters have a display of different kinds of appliances. Appliance ads in the *Ostomy Quarterly,* a visit to a pharmacy or surgical supply house which stocks appliances, or word of mouth from other ostomates can all be helpful. However, considering how important a properly fitted appliance is, it would be a blessing if all ostomates could have the advantage of advice from an ET or from another health professional with wide experience of ostomies.

When Don Binder had his ileostomy in 1959, there weren't any ETs around to advise him. After a number of wild goose chases, "We went to a surgical supply dealer who showed us an appliance that didn't require cement. We bought it and I immediately put it on. Then we went to a supermarket, and as I was pushing the cart I felt the trickle on my leg. We later discovered that what we had bought was a colostomy irrigating dome which had no protection for the skin. The salesperson didn't know the difference nor did I. Fortunately, that doesn't happen very often these days."

Basically, appliances divide themselves into disposable (which are discarded after one use, usually a few days), and reusable pouches (washed and then used again, many times). Using disposables regularly costs more money but saves time. When it's time to change the appliance, the ostomate simply throws the used pouch in the trash (after wrapping it securely in aluminum foil or other covering).

The ostomate who relies on reusable pouches usually has two or three. While one is being worn, another is being soaked, dried, and aired. Special cleaning-soaking solutions, which clean, deodorize, and maintain ostomy appliances, can be purchased from the appliance supplier. (For the urostomate, there are specific products to clean appliances and dissolve crystals left by urine.) After soaking the appliance, ostomates can use an appliance cleaning brush, or a baby-bottle brush to scrub the inside of the pouch.

Appliances also come in one-piece or two-piece styles. A one-piece appliance has an adhesive disc, bonded to the plastic pouch, which attaches to the skin directly. Many ostomates prefer

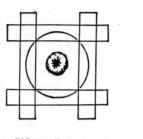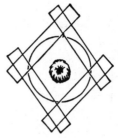

PICTURE FRAME   DIAMOND

PUTTING ON TAPE

porous tape around the faceplate to hold the appliance more securely to the skin.

Some appliances are available with a belt; some are not. If a belt is worn, it should be positioned around the hips even with the stoma, and there should be room for two fingers to slip easily under the belt. Occasional use of a belt (during active sports, for instance) should cause no problems, or only very minor ones.

In a two-piece appliance, a separate faceplate is adhered to the skin, often with a cement which is applied thinly to faceplate and skin and then allowed to dry thoroughly before the faceplate is attached. A pouch is then fastened to this. For some ostomates with special problems, like a flush ileostomy stoma which requires a convex faceplate, the two-piece appliance may be the only kind which works well. Other ostomates may find this more comfortable, more secure, or more protective. (Athletes in contact sports may prefer a fairly sturdy faceplate for this reason.) Some people may simply have used a two-piece appliance for years, and see no reason to change.

The best time to change an appliance is when the ostomy is least active. For urostomates, although drainage is constant, the stoma may be less active early in the morning before breakfast. Cotton or tissue in an empty pill bottle with an opening the size of

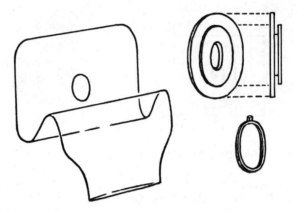

Two-piece appliance has separate faceplate, usually constructed of a sturdy material. Pouch is attached to a faceplate, using a two-faced adhesive seal, cement, or locking device supplied by manufacturer. Two-piece appliance pictured is for an ileostomy; other ostomates also use this type.

the stoma, can catch drainage and keep the skin around the stoma dry while the appliance is being changed; a tampon will do the same. For many ileostomates with unpredictable ostomies, tissue over the stoma is useful while the skin around the stoma is being prepared for a fresh appliance.

Until recent years, odor was an almost insurmountable problem for ostomates, a frequent source of whispers and non-acceptance. Now, thanks to advances in appliance materials and more trustworthy deodorants, odor is seldom a problem, although it may take a little trial and error to find the best protection.

Cleanliness is the basis of any attack on unwanted odors—baths or showers and well-cleaned reusable appliances, or new disposables. Appliances are now built to hold gas, sometimes a source of odor, until there's privacy to release it—either through an opening at the bottom or through a built-in gas release valve.

Although many appliances are now so odor-proof that no deodorant is necessary, a number of ostomy suppliers offer effective deodorants. These are usually in liquid form. A few drops in the pouch at each opening, rinsing, or change suffice. Some ostomates depend on oral deodorants — bismuth compounds taken in pill form on a regular daily basis. (While these are effective, bismuth is a heavy metal with possible side effects; its use should be discussed with the doctor or ET.) The ET also has expert advice on the best ways to deal with odor if special problems arise.

From experience, ostomates discover that some foods increase odor in feces or urine. This is a highly individual matter, so a little detective work is necessary. Parsley and yogurt, used liberally in the diet, are recommended by many as good natural ways to control odor.

Appliances can be expensive. Medicare, Medicaid, and some insurance programs cover ostomy supplies. To insure proper credit, appliance products should be described as "prosthetic appliances." If money is a problem, the ostomate may decide on reusable appliances rather than disposable ones, or may improvise with different kinds of plastic bags or other materials.

It's worthwhile for every ostomate to find a pharmacy or appliance supply source which is really interested in ostomates and well-informed. Some of the large mail order firms which have been in business a long time are able and willing to offer personalized advice. For those with a special problem, some companies specialize in custom appliances.

The good old days? They weren't all that good for people with ostomies — and the appliance companies, which have produced booklets, slide shows and films on ostomy care, along with a continuing stream of new appliances and skin care products, can take much of the credit for the enormous strides forward in a very few years.

Virginia Pearce looks back a few decades at the days after her ileostomy: "Several *weeks* after surgery the long awaited appliance arrived . . . a COLOSTOMY pouch with a wire frame that protruded out about an inch. When I was first told about this 'ileostomy' and having to wear a 'bag', I decided that my life would be spent in maternity smocks, and when THAT appliance was presented to me, I *knew* I was going to look pregnant for the next 30 or 40 years.

"But the worst was yet to come. This pouch had no bottom opening, a three-inch stoma opening and was held on by belts and buckles, no cement or skin barrier. When I sat up in the wheelchair my tummy was concave (hard to believe now) and warm, brown fluid trickled down my abdomen . . . ah! the good old days!

"Determined there must be a *better* appliance somewhere, I got a pass from the hospital, hired a cab, and went to the biggest surgical supply house in Salt Lake City.

"The sales person showed me the only alternative appliance he had. There was a metal ring (with a two inch opening) and over the ring you put latex rubber pouches which went inside a white satin cover. The purpose of the lovely satin cover was to keep the thin rubber pouch from elongating as it filled up. The appliance had a wide belt and buckles — no cement. Very often when you sat down, with a partially filled pouch, everything 'pooched up' and over, and there was that nice brown stain again! . . . .

"Ah, the good old days!"

CHANGING AN APPLIANCE

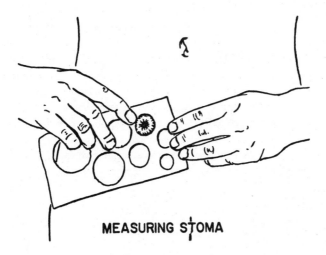

MEASURING STOMA

1. MEASURING STOMA TO GET CORRECT APPLIANCE SIZE. Appliance manufacturers supply measuring devices for the stoma. To find the right size stoma opening for the appliance, the ostomate finds the smallest cutout ring which fits comfortably around the stoma without touching it. This gives the stoma room to expand slightly when it is discharging waste, but permits the appliance to cover most of the skin around the stoma. The distance across the cutout ring will be the size for a pre-cut appliance (a 1½-inch stoma ring means a 1½-inch appliance)—or it can be used as a pattern if the ostomate is cutting his/her own opening. The ostomate with an irregularly-shaped stoma cuts out a pattern to fit the stoma.

The initial measuring is done soon after surgery, quite frequently during the first weeks while the stoma size is changing, and once in a while after that, especially if there is a weight change.

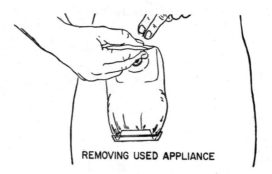

REMOVING USED APPLIANCE

2. REMOVING USED APPLIANCE. This is done *gently* to protect the skin around the stoma. First the appliance is emptied. Then, while one hand removes the appliance, the other hand supports the skin around the stoma. If cement has been used to adhere the appliance to the skin, the correct solvent is applied with a cotton-tip applicator to the area at the edge of the appliance; when the cement has been dissolved in that area, the loosened section of the appliance is eased from the skin. This process is repeated as necessary. The soiled appliance is set aside.

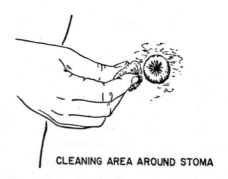

CLEANING AREA AROUND STOMA

3. CLEANING AREA AROUND STOMA. A shower, bath or sponge bath with warm water cleans the area well. The skin is washed gently, not rubbed. If mild soap is used, it must be rinsed off completely. The skin is then blotted completely dry. If the stoma continues discharging during the cleaning process, a tampon or a pill bottle the size of the stoma can catch any waste.

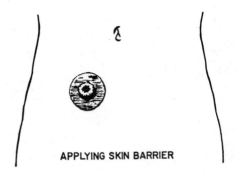

APPLYING SKIN BARRIER

4. APPLYING SKIN BARRIER. Many ostomates rely on some kind of commercial product to protect the skin around the stoma. These products, which come as a pliable gum (either as a pre-cut ring or as a sheet), paste, powder, spray, creme, or liquid, protect the skin right up to the stoma. Directions for each product will be on the container.

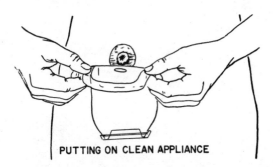

PUTTING ON CLEAN APPLIANCE

5. PUTTING ON CLEAN APPLIANCE. If there is an opening at the bottom of the appliance, it is closed. The ostomate slowly peels away the backing paper from the appliance seal as he/she attaches the appliance to the abdomen carefully and smoothly, with no air pockets. If a cement is used, a *thin* coat is applied to both the appliance faceplate and to a circle of skin around the stoma slightly larger than the area the faceplate will cover. The cement is allowed to dry for several minutes before the appliance is attached. In the case of a two-piece appliance, the separate faceplate is adhered to the skin; the pouch is then secured to the faceplate.

Appliances and the Skin They Touch   1 1 3

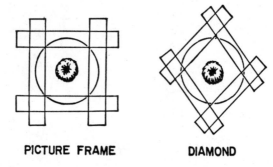

PICTURE FRAME   **DIAMOND**

6. PUTTING ON TAPE. A porous tape can be used—picture-frame fashion—around the edges of the appliance faceplate. Some ostomates use a belt, which is put on around the hips at the level of the stoma, loosely enough so that two fingers can be slipped between belt and skin.

CHAPTER 13 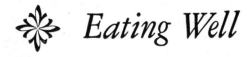 *Eating Well*

*. . . she opened it, and found in it a very small cake, on which
the words "EAT ME" were beautifully marked in currants.
"Well, I'll eat it," said Alice, "and if it makes me larger,
I can reach the key; and if it makes me smaller,
I can creep under the door. . . .*
Lewis Carroll, *Alice in Wonderland*

"Curiouser and curiouser," cried Alice — and people with
ostomies, confused about what they can and should eat, might
well echo the bewildered lass. Someone says, "Eat what your
doctor says." But then the doctor says, "Eat what you want." What
to do?

If the new ostomate is perplexed, trying to juggle protein and
"residue" and electrolytes and calories and dollars, he's not alone.
"The only thing I can count on now," said a non-ostomate, "is that
if I like some food, an expert will say 'It's bad for you'!" Or it costs
too much.

In the midst of this muddle, a few points remain clear. The
ostomate needs to be well nourished. Surgery hasn't changed the
physical (or the emotional) need for good food.

For the first week or two after surgery, the question of what's for
dinner tomorrow remains academic, and more than a little dull.
Until the digestive tract settles down, the new ostomate is stuck

with bland, *low residue* food. Then, as the sense of adventure regenerates, the longing for greener pastures—or at least a leaf of lettuce—returns.

Fortunately, the greener pastures are usually within reach. Most ostomates, after they recuperate, can eat most foods.

Eating well is one of the real rewards for the ileostomate with surgery for inflammatory bowel disease, who's been banished to bland cereal and applesauce too long, and who needs to rebuild a scrawny figure. Whenever cancer is involved (as it often is with colostomies and urostomies), eating well is one of the best kinds of medicine, for both body and spirit. And—whatever the major surgery—food's the real lifeline for getting the body strong and fit again.

First things first: how do we become well nourished?

The body needs raw materials for the processes necessary for life — and it needs a steady source of them. Food supplies these building blocks for energy, and for tissue growth and repair in the body. It also provides some of the chemical regulators which the body needs to change these raw materials into energy and tissue. To do all this, the body needs six different kinds of *nutrients*, or specific components of food: carbohydrates, proteins, fats, vitamins, minerals, and water.

Most foods combine all or several of these components. Milk, for instance, contains all six (including some of the vitamins and minerals, although not all). So does a cucumber, but the amounts are less, and the proportions are different. Putting these foods together so that we get enough of each nutrient to keep the body operating — and there are endless ways to do it — is how we nourish ourselves. Thanks to the variety, we can add foods we like, subtract those we can't afford, substitute intelligently (grains, nuts, milk, and eggs for meat, for example), and still emerge with healthy, delicious, affordable fare.

A few years ago, nutritionists figured out a fairly simple way for people to put together a healthy, well-balanced diet without having to count each gram of carbohydrate, every milligram of vitamin B-2. If adults eat or drink two 8-ounce servings of milk (or the equivalent in milk products), two 3-ounce servings of meat or high protein foods (fish, eggs, nuts, soybean, for instance), four helpings of fruit or vegetables (1/2 cup cooked vegetable or one fresh orange is one serving), and four servings of cereal and grains (one slice of bread equals one serving) each day, they probably get the basic nutrients they need. There are other ways to put together a healthy diet. Many people, for example, concerned with the amount of animal protein and fat in the diet, work out their meals around combinations of lower protein non-animal foods which, eaten together, give the body the protein it needs.

Some ostomates have special needs for three of the nutrients: vitamins, minerals, and water.

Many nutritionists believe that a healthy, varied selection of foods provides all the vitamins (the chemical regulators the body needs in tiny amounts to keep running smoothly) most people need. There is one exception for some ileostomates and a few urostomates (those with ileal conduits involving the very end of the ileum): vitamin B-12, which is absorbed in the section of intestine where small and large bowel join. Even when all of this is removed during surgery, many ostomates seem to have little trouble, but some may need a B-12 injection every few months. Loss of appetite and decreased energy may result from a deficiency; a check with the doctor is in order.

Electrolyte is a common term in ostomy language. An electrolyte is an electrical charge which plays a big role in how the body functions. These charges come from minerals (such as sodium, potassium and calcium) dissolved in the body fluids.

When the large intestine, which absorbs a large amount of water into the body, is missing, the water goes directly through the digestive tract, and carries with it those electrolytes which are dissolved in it. Sodium is not usually a problem, since the typical American diet contains far more salt than the body can use, but potassium and other electrolytes sometimes wash out faster from this salty internal sea than the body can replenish them.

Potassium-rich foods, like bananas, oranges, prunes, and

tomatoes (and there are many more; lists are readily available), solve the problem most of the time; potassium also comes as a liquid or powder supplement, to be used with medical supervision only. During a short bout of diarrhea or vomiting, or during very hot weather, ostomates can replace unusual losses with Gatorade® or a homemade recipe. (One calls for 1 teaspoon each salt and baking soda, 4 teaspoons white Karo® syrup, and 1 6-ounce can frozen orange juice in enough water to make 1 quart —drinking ½ cup every hour.) If the problem continues, medical help is essential.

People don't think of water as food, but it, too, is an essential nutrient, needed in constant supply. With the short-circuit in their water-absorbing colon, ileostomates and colostomates with loose stools require even more water, and food with large water content, than most people do; the kidneys, which do most of the regulating of water and electrolytes in the body, compensate for some of the loss. Drinking more water does *not* increase bowel output. Ileostomates need to keep drinking so that the substances that cause kidney stones keep flushing out of the kidneys. Urostomates also need to keep drinking so that any bacteria that may cause kidney infection keep washing out of the conduit.

Many Americans—with and without ostomies—worry about their weight. Everyone has a favorite diet, whether it's a bedraggled carrot and lettuce leaf smorgasbord or a melon mania. With ileostomates, especially, the problem may sneak up. Before surgery, they fought desperately for each pound; suddenly, after surgery, bulges and double-chins appear. Other ostomates may be trying to gain weight, and they too will be counting *calories*, those measures of heat (energy) released when a food is processed in the body; 3500 calories beyond what the body needs to maintain itself means one pound of extra weight; this extra fat comes from carbohydrates, fats, protein, and alcohol.

The common sense approach to dieting starts with making food really *work* in the body. Most foods contain several of the six nutrient types, so that they are doing other things for the body *besides* creating calories of energy. The "junk foods," on the other hand—the candy, the cookies from refined sugar, the alcohol— provide calories and that's about all. We still have to eat all the rest of the foods, which incidentally also contain calories, to meet our bodies' needs.

Most nutritionists agree that although the body needs fats, it doesn't need nearly as many of them as the typical diet includes. Since fats are concentrated sources of calories, they are a leverage food for losing or gaining weight.

Fiber—also called roughage or residue or bulk—is the new darling of the nutritionists. Fiber is an undigestible carbohydrate (like bran and parts of fruits and vegetables). It contributes nothing to human nutrition, but acts as a sponge in the intestine, soaking up water to soften the stool and speed it on its way. In general, a low residue diet tends to be constipating. On the other hand, the digestive tracts of most ileostomates can't handle a very high fiber diet, laced with large quantities of bran.

Many ostomates do very nicely by avoiding both extremes and aiming for moderate residue, with some whole grain breads and cereals, and some raw or partially cooked fruits and vegetables. Some ileostomates tolerate this amount of bulk with ease, or are willing to cope with more frequent emptying of an appliance.

Most ostomates can eat most things. But it's an individual matter. Considering how important eating well is, it would be great if there were ileostomy diets, colostomy diets, and urostomy diets, all ready to hand out along with any other hospital discharge material. Unfortunately, there's a lot more trial and error than that.

One ileostomate, from Coos Bay, Oregon, reported: "When I had my ileostomy, my surgeon told me I could eat anything that agreed with me. After so many years of diet because of ulcerative colitis, I could hardly believe my ears! However, that little phrase, 'that agreed with me,' was the joker."

She checked with other ileostomates and found that everyone had a few foods to avoid — but they were different foods for different individuals: "One eats applesauce to stop the 'runs' while I eat applesauce if I need something to act as a mild laxative."

"Our systems are so different, no one, not even a doctor, can give you a diet list and expect it to work for you ... as for an ileostomy diet, there is no such thing! We find out, sometimes the hard way, if we have eaten something we shouldn't."

It's best to go slowly after surgery, adding a small amount of a new food at a time and then waiting 24-48 hours to see what happens. Even if a food disagrees the first time, it can be tried again a few weeks later, perhaps in a smaller amount. And if peanuts don't work, maybe peanut butter will. The blender can make foods that are too fibrous more tolerable.

Many ileostomates and some colostomates avoid, or eat sparingly, foods with a large amount of *cellulose,* a kind of fiber found in popcorn, coconut, stringy celery, shells of peas, and such Chinese vegetables as bean sprouts and bamboo shoots. These, along with granola-type cereals and nuts, especially when taken in large amounts, and hastily chewed, are the villains in most food blockages. In a blockage, the bowel clogs up with undigested food, the ostomy stops functioning, and the abdomen starts cramping.

Most blockages resolve themselves quickly. First step is to put on a soft, disposable appliance with a large stoma opening, so that the swelling stoma is not constricted. Then, simple remedies can be tried, like changing position or relaxing in the bath. (If the ostomy doesn't start working again after two hours or so, it's time for medical help.)

There'd be far fewer blockages if all ostomates were better chewers, but.... One of the food Messiahs around the turn of the century was a gentleman named Fletcher, who tried to sell "Fletcherism" — chewing every bite of food 30 times. Probably ileostomates who revived Fletcherism could eat anything. On the other hand, such a safe and cautious approach might spoil the fun for people like our friend Rachel, who delights in calling a dish of popcorn and a glass of lemonade lunch, just to prove she can!

Ostomates have no monopoly on passing gas. But ileostomates

and colostomates probably worry about it more because it comes through the abdomen—and involuntarily—rather than through the rectum, and more voluntarily.

The cause and the solution probably vary with different kinds of ostomies. The "gas" expelled by the ostomate may be swallowed air. Eating slowly, sipping rather than gulping drinks, giving up chewing gum can reduce air swallowing.

Onions, cabbage, baked beans, cucumbers are notorious gas-causers for many people, with or without ostomies. A number of reports suggest that too high an intake of refined sugar and flour (in cookies and other sweets) may lead to gas for some people. A little detective work may be in order, and a willingness to give up a problem food. Observing when gas occurs, and remembering what was eaten in the last several hours, provide the clues. Ostomates swear by their favorite remedies: buttermilk is one, or yogurt (preferably the plain variety, flavored with fresh fruits at home).

If the offender is the "trapped gas" dear to TV commercials, anything which hastens peristalsis will hasten relief. A small meal, half a cup of coffee, exercise, or massaging the abdomen may help. Some use over-the-counter nostrums, but it's wise to consult a doctor before trying this. Going too long between meals is a major cause of gas; more frequent meals can be the answer.

Meanwhile, a bit of privacy until the gas is released may be comforting, since gas may have a strong odor. The release of gas can be controlled through the bottom of the appliance, a pinhole (subsequently covered with non-porous tape) or a built-in gas release valve.

Some ostomates have special diet needs. The book *Nutrition for the Cancer Patient*, by Rosenbaum, Stitt, Drasin, and Rosenbaum (Bull Publishing Co., 1980), has concrete suggestions, especially for those undergoing chemotherapy or radiation. People with ostomies who also have other medical problems, such as high blood pressure or diabetes, can learn about their particular diets with the help of a dietitian.

The U.S. Government publishes a wealth of free or low-cost

brochures and booklets about nutrition, meal planning, thrifty recipes, and similar topics. A postcard to the Consumer Information Center, Dept. 648G, Pueblo, Colorado 81009, will bring a complete list of publications.

Our bodies depend on good food. Our spirits, no less, are nourished, whether by the hearty stew shared with family, the romantic candle-lit dinner with a loved one, or the meal prepared with care by the person living alone, and served with a vase of daisies on the tray.

Food is an adventure, and a delight. From time to time, it's even worth breaking a rule or two. That's how our friend Ann feels about it. Says Ann, an ileostomate for many years: "I *love* cucumbers, always have. They bring back summer . . . and picnics when I was a kid. Sure, I know that cucumbers don't like me much, that I'll be emptying my appliance all the time if I eat one.

"But every once in awhile . . . it's worth it!"

CHAPTER 14   ✤   *Catnaps,*
Strolls, and Good Belly
Laughs

It's time to go, to run, to rise up, to fling open the window, thaw
the blood, prance high in the wet grass—to shout and feel and
seek new rootholds in the nourishing earth.
William Hedgepeth

When Neanderthal Ned ventured out of his cave some
thousands of years ago — and found himself face-to-face with a
large and furious beast—his body responded. Ned's adrenals, tiny
glands nestled above each kidney, sent an instant chemical
message to the rest of the body: emergency! Ned's heart raced,
pumping blood laced with oxygen through ready vessels to lungs,
arms, legs, shunting it away from the rest of the body during this
crisis. If the beast was very large, and maybe a little slow and
nearsighted, Ned took to his heels, fleeing danger. Or, strength
surging, Ned faced and fought the beast. The crisis resolved
quickly. Sometimes Ned won, sometimes the beast.

Modern man lives in different circumstances — with the same
body. Evolving over millions of years to survive short

emergencies, the body has not progressed (or regressed) to fit the way many of us live now. Faced with any kind of stress, or change in its equilibrium, it reacts in the same all-out fashion: blood vessels constrict, heart pounds, skin perspires to cope with the increased heat of racing blood, digestive tract slows to a halt, sexual energies dissolve.

But, except for the rare emergency (like grabbing a child out of the path of an onrushing car), we usually face chronic rather than acute stress. And often we can neither fight nor flee. Instead we continue to face the same stressful situations day after day, month after month: a demanding job, a difficult (and unchangeable) employer, daily traffic jams, inflation, illness, worries about those dear to us. All too often we can neither resolve the problem nor get away from it.

Hans Selye, a Canadian physiologist who accidentally discovered what happened to adrenal glands under continuing stress, led the way to a whole new perspective on health and illness. He considers stress "the spice of life," a good and necessary thing in our lives — within reason. We cannot change or grow without stress: "Since stress is associated with all types of activity, we could avoid most of it only by never doing anything. Who would enjoy a life of no runs, no hits, no errors?"

But constant stress does peculiar and devastating things to the body. Blood vessels, constricted by adrenalin, forget how to relax, perhaps leading to high blood pressure. With the action shunted away from it to the emergency centers of the body, the digestive tract slows down—and a multi-million-dollar laxative industry springs up.

And the poor adrenals, expected to cope with never-ending crises, grow weary. Increasingly sturdy research points to a connection between serious disease and an overload of stress. Our bodies deal successfully every day with disease-causers: bacteria, viruses, carcinogens (cancer-causing substances). As long as our defenses are strong, we don't get sick. But, with unremitting stress, the body's protective systems grow exhausted or confused.

Invaders slip past—bringing perhaps just a cold, perhaps cancer. Or the body starts seeing invaders where there aren't any and begins attacking itself, as appears to happen in some of the inflammatory bowel diseases.

If we get the message, along with our ostomy surgery, either that we've been facing too much stress, or that our system for coping with it needs an overhaul, then we can seize the chance to become healthier and happier than we've ever been. (Obviously, the disease, the surgery and the new ostomy add to the stress load, temporarily.) Knowing there's a problem is the first step toward solving it.

When our friend Helen was recovering from throat cancer, for example, her doctor insisted that she cut down the amount of stress in her life. That's a tall order, but Helen took it seriously. She simplified here, and delegated authority there. She described to us one change—small, but telling: as a bit of "self-discipline," she had gotten into the habit of always swallowing the large number of pills prescribed for her *before* yielding to the demands of her bladder, however urgent. Now the bladder wins!

If we listen to them, our bodies can often tell us things we wouldn't dare to admit to ourselves. Kathy, a non-ostomate, confesses: "I always knew I didn't like my boss — but I didn't realize *how* furious I was at him. Finally I put two and two together and figured out that the only time my bowel wasn't on the warpath was when he was sick or on vacation—then I knew I had to make a change."

Many an ostomate could echo her. Since the digestive tract (and even the urinary tract, sometimes) turns sluggish or starts racing partly in response to the stress messages of the body, our ostomies warn us that maybe some quiet moments are overdue. How relaxed we are certainly isn't the only factor in making an ostomy behave happily — but it's a *big* one.

Some stresses we can't avoid. But some we can. The Serenity Prayer (p. 44)—changing what can be changed, accepting what can't be changed, and knowing the difference—says it best. Often, if we can *space* or *postpone* the avoidable stresses, we can manage the unavoidable ones.

Sometimes we need help. For comfort and reassurance as we move through unavoidable stresses, family, friends, doctor, and clergymen can lend a hand. Sometimes, with personal counseling, we learn that we are putting ourselves under intolerable stress to maintain a particular image of ourselves. When we can let go of that "Superman" or "Perfect Mother" (or whatever) image, we find out that we *can* avoid some of those "unavoidable" stresses. And if we can let go the burdens of yesterday and tomorrow, we are free to enjoy the pleasures of today.

Neanderthal Ned faced his share of stress. But if he survived the encounter with large-and-furious beast, he had a chance to loll about the cave a bit, chew a few berries, and have a pleasant dinner of ex-furious beast. Even if we can't change our stress load, we can give our bodies a chance to rest up, to recuperate from the arrows of daily life.

When Norman Cousins, editor of *The Saturday Review,* heard his acute illness diagnosed as a life-threatening disease in 1964, he searched back over the past hectic months for possible causes. It became more and more clear to him that an exhausted adrenal system, worn out by both acute and chronic stress without relief, was a big factor. Since there was no known treatment for the disease, Cousins decided, with his doctor's encouragement, to bolster the tired adrenals, using his own therapy of belly laughs and vitamin C. Comedy film clips, anthologies of humor, took the place of pain shots. As he tells it in *Anatomy of an Illness* (Norton, 1979), he "made the joyous discovery that ten minutes of genuine belly laughter had an anesthetic effect and would give me at least two hours of pain-free sleep." The disease retreated.

Exercise is another natural relaxer. In fact, since our body's response to stress equips it to flee or to fight, running — or walking, or in fact any vigorous activity—is ideal. It's what our body wants us to do. A brisk walk around the block clears not only the mind but the body.

Slow deep breathing, too, holds special magic for ostomates. As part of exercise, or on its own, it gets rid of some of the chemical residue of the body's response to stress. And it feels so good. Taking slow deep breaths, we fill the lungs. It's an ancient technique for relaxing, cheaper and safer than tranquilizers or alcohol.

Sometimes we have a hobby or favorite activity that lets the tension slip away like an ebbing tide. As we pick up a trowel in the garden, or sit down at the piano, or take a stitch in the embroidery, we can feel a gentle relaxation flow over us. Doing something for ourselves—whether it's listening to a favorite piece of music or reading a good book or talking to a friend—revives us. Or maybe it's just doing something completely different from our usual job—perhaps working at a hospital as a volunteer once a week—that recharges us.

And then there's sleep. "That we are not much sicker and much madder than we are," writes Aldous Huxley, "is due exclusively to that most blessed and blessing of all natural graces, sleep."

Whether it's a catnap or a full eight hours, sleep refreshes. Sleep restores. And it is also a subtle barometer of how well we are dealing with the stress in our lives.

Perhaps Neanderthal Ned slipped into sleep as effortlessly as a kitten does. But with our different kind of stress, we don't always sleep soundly and easily. Surgery can be a springboard for addiction to sleeping pills; it's easy—and sometimes necessary— to resort to this chemical aid in the hospital when pain, unfamiliar surroundings, hospital noise, lack of exercise, and anxiety take their toll. But over long periods, sleeping pills are not good.

There are better answers. Some exercise before bedtime, a warm bath, a good (but not too exciting) book, a glass of warm milk, are all natural soporifics, lulling us to natural sleep. A bedtime routine (even without the teddy bear tuck-in!) readies us. A comfortable bed helps.

But the core of the matter is relaxation. No matter how

comfortable the bed, no matter how tired we are, there is no way for us to sleep peacefully with taut muscles, clenched jaws and a racing mind. Luckily, we can learn how to relax; it's a skill we can draw on during the day as well as at bedtime.

Many people find one of the meditation techniques effective. By concentrating on one word or phrase for a time, at regular intervals, they slip into serene relaxation. Picturing an appealing scene—perhaps a secluded, sun-drenched beach—relaxes others. Some people find that praying—laying troubles in the lap of a higher being—is all they need.

Or we can approach relaxation from another angle and relax the body physically. Although it may seem like putting the cart before the horse, the relaxed body seems to draw the mind with it.

One method for relaxing the body involves first tensing a small group of muscles (like the arm), becoming aware of just how it feels, and then slowly, consciously, releasing the tension, feeling it flow away. Starting with legs and arms and trunk, one works up to shoulders, neck, jaw. What surprises most of us when we're learning how to relax is finding out just how tense we are most of the time. It takes a while to learn how to unknot those muscles at will. There are some quick first-aid techniques for relaxing. Shaking an arm or leg, for instance, unkinks those taut muscles.

Relaxation classes, books on relaxing, stress reduction clinics, professional massage, sophisticated technology (like bio-feedback, in which a person learning to relax hears a tone indicating how taut or relaxed a muscle is and gradually learns to sustain the "relaxed tone")—all are ways of helping a tense world unwind.

Unless we're lumps, we face stress in our lives. So probably we all could use some healthy way of handling that stress. Some kind of relaxation belongs in our daily lives.

We each find our own ways. Nadine Stair wrote about her ways —at age 85:

"If I had to live my life over again, I'd dare to make more mistakes next time.

I'd relax.

I would limber up.

I would be sillier than I have been this trip.

I would take fewer things seriously.

I would take more chances.

I would take more trips. I would climb more mountains, swim more rivers.

I would eat more ice cream and less beans.

I would perhaps have more actual troubles, but I'd have fewer imaginary ones.

You see, I'm one of those people who live seriously and sanely hour after hour, day after day.

Oh, I've had my moments. And if I had it to do over again, I'd have more of them.

In fact, I'd try to have nothing else, just moments, one after another, instead of living so many years ahead of each day.

I've been one of those persons who never goes anywhere without a thermometer, a hot water bottle, a raincoat and a parachute.

If I had it to do again I would travel lighter than I have.

If I had to live my life over, I would start barefoot earlier in the spring, and stay that way later in fall.

I would go to more dances.

I would ride more merry-go-rounds.

I would pick more daisies."

CHAPTER 15 ❁ *You're Looking Great*

Thoreau warned us: "Beware of all enterprises that require new clothes, and not rather a new wearer of clothes."

Thoreau had a point, or rather two, and both ring bells with ostomates. We are new wearers of clothes, given new life by a surgical detour. And while the enterprise may not *require* new clothes (except for maybe a bathing suit with a slightly different cut), an ostomy is a grand excuse for a little shopping.

In the beginning, shuffling down the hall in a baggy hospital gown, dragging a reluctant IV stand in my wake, I found it hard to believe I'd ever look really good again or be able to wear anything but shapeless sacks or rumpled bathrobes. In theory, especially after meeting a UOA visitor or two, smartly dressed in snug-fitting clothes, I knew it could be done. But! Incision tender, abdomen puffy, stoma still almost a stranger and covered with that unfamiliar post-op appliance, perineal wound draining and tweaking like a toothache, I felt uncomfortable, awkward, and unattractive. Looking great? Nonsense! As my mother used to say, I looked as if I were sent for and couldn't come.

It's a little like getting back to normal after having a baby. The woman who tries to wear her pre-pregnancy slacks home from the hospital after delivery finds it just doesn't work—at first. A few weeks later, they may fit fine.

As the incision healed, the stoma shrank, and pain became something I could barely remember, I began to notice clothing ads in the morning paper. And to remember how smart Ann and Dorothy looked. Person after person has reported disbelief—and the beginning of hope—when they met their first UOA visitor. Whatever else they forget, they all seem to remember that the visitor was well dressed! As one ostomate reported in the Metro Maryland newsletter, "In less than two hours, a lovely lady entered my room, beautifully dressed, and announced who she was. From that day on everything improved. Her image has been with me these past four years."

Clothes that look good and feel good are an important bridge back to the world, one way of mending a bruised body image and moving ahead from *patient* to *person*. A well-cut sports coat or a new haircut is a flag being raised with the message: "I'm not licked!"

An ostomy seldom limits anyone's clothing horizons; sometimes it expands them. As a result, people with an ostomy are perhaps a little better dressed than the average person. They've learned that looking good is important to their own morale, even if no one sees but the mirror. Looking good also brings positive feedback. I discovered that when a friend said, "Wow! You look great!" I felt better. And when—instead of offering sympathy or chicken soup—they said, "Let's go out to lunch," I was almost mended.

Few ostomates are ready for modeling assignments the first few weeks or even months after surgery. (I never was, but that had nothing to do with surgery.) Abdominal tenderness and a still sore perineal area make looser than usual clothes comfortable. For women, this may mean wraparound skirts instead of pants suits, and A-line dresses or gaudy caftans instead of snug sheaths. Until one gets used to a changed body, overblouses or shirts worn outside pants offer welcome reassurance. In this period, until they're sure their new control systems don't leak, many ostomates prefer prints or plaids to solid colors, so any small accident would go unnoticed.

Night gowns (or night shirts) feel better than pajamas. For both men and women, suspenders may be more tolerable temporarily than belts. Both may wish to change underwear types, switching to underpants which come above or below the stoma and not right on top of it. For underpants, cotton absorbs perspiration better than synthetic fabrics, yet need not look like great aunt Minnie's winter drawers. If the perineal wound is still draining, sanitary mini-pads affixed to underpants may be used.

After convalescence, there are few limits. Appliances are now so slim they don't show under snug clothing (with the possible exception of thin, clinging jerseys). Light-weight girdles for women and supports for men are optional (unless the doctor orders them). Tight girdles or belts which rub the stoma should be avoided.

Thanks to new flexibility in fashion, there are usually enough variations in style in any season so it's easy to find something that's good looking, comfortable and as fashionable as one cares to be. If Bill Blass hasn't designed just the right thing this season, Halston or someone else probably has.

For ideas on looking good with an ostomy, nothing beats attending the local UOA meeting (or, a little later, a regional or national conference). My first meeting astounded me. I guess I'd expected a roomful of gloomy Joes and grim Gerties, all feeling sorry for themselves. But I was wrong, and I remember clearly my first impression: "These *can't* be people with ostomies. They look too good. . . ." Perhaps they weren't all fashion plates, but they cared about their appearance, and about grooming. They knew the image they presented to the world was important, not only personally, but to new ostomates and the world in general.

In addition to expecting a dreary and depressing group at that first UOA meeting, I think I'd been apprehensive about odor.

Could an ostomate deal with this? Apparently they could, for all my nose remembers is the good smell of coffee brewing for the laughter-filled social hour after the meeting.

If the budget permits, ostomy surgery provides a fine excuse for getting something new and pleasing to wear. New ileostomates may want to hold off major clothing purchases for a bit until weight stabilizes. Before surgery, the problem was keeping weight up; now everything tastes so good, it may be hard to keep the extra pounds off.

However therapeutic a new wardrobe may be, medical insurance doesn't pay for it. There are alternatives. If money is scarce, ingenuity needn't be. Changing a collar style, shortening sleeves, adding a little embroidery, converting a tired dress to a fresh new skirt—there may be more in the closet than we think. Another possibility is a visit to a local thrift shop or a garage sale.

With new energy and more dependable bodies, ostomates may need new kinds of clothes to follow new paths—a jogging suit, a business-like dress for a new job, drip-dry separates for travel, clothes for dancing or swimming or tennis. Or even a wedding dress....

Vicki Cunning of Irving, Texas, found herself not only enjoying new clothes after her surgery, but modeling them as part of her job: "Suddenly it was zero hour and we were dressed. And ready? Well, maybe not completely ready inside, but it was too late now! Lights! Music! Action! My first outfit had buttons down the front. I was shaking so hard when I got off the stage someone had to unbutton it. I seemed to get braver (they had told us that we would), because the more that I went on the easier it got. We danced rather than just walked up and down that runway! Me, with an ileostomy! I was a model!"

Children with ostomies don't need special clothes—just ones they like. Those who have surgery to control dribbling urine rejoice in a world without wet pants or diapers and are free to wear clothes they couldn't risk before, including Little League uniforms and ballet costumes. As for any children, easy-care, comfortable clothes are best for school and play, with something special for big occasions.

For thousands of ostomates, the prognosis is excellent. For some, it's not that good. Our friend Trudy taught us that even a somewhat gloomy diagnosis is no reason to wear dreary clothes. During radiation and after, she lost a lot of weight. She'd always been proud of her figure and found her new scrawniness depressing, so she went shopping. In addition to an apricot plush housecoat that caught her eye, she got some soft cotton blouses with full sleeves, a skirt with a little more fullness, a jumper cut wide enough so she could wear turtlenecks under it, and a couple of gaudy kimonos.

"The new clothes weren't an extravagance, really. Wearing them, I feel better about myself and it's surprising how often friends say, 'You're looking great!' They've stopped treating me like a thin china cup, and I'm enjoying each day more."

Among people with ostomies, some favor soft worn jeans, some are never caught in anything but the latest fashion, and there are thousands and thousands in between. In one way or another, though, clothes are a useful shorthand, telling the world, "An ostomy is OK—and so am I!"

CHAPTER 16 ❧ *What About Sex?*

Male and female he created them. . . .
Genesis

Some things are better than sex, and some are worse, but there's
nothing exactly like it.
W. C. Fields

From birth to death, we are sexual persons — and ostomy surgery doesn't change that. So it's natural to wonder about sex after surgery: "Can I?" "Will anyone want me?" "Can I give and receive pleasure?"

For most people, sex can be as good as it was before, or even better (if surgery follows years of severe ulcerative colitis, for instance). People with ostomies date, fall in love, marry and have children. For some, there may be problems, temporary or permanent; even then, there are possible remedies and alternatives.

We bring all of ourselves to sex—our beliefs, expectations and experiences. Whether it's part of a loving long-term relationship or a shorter exploration, sex is a special kind of communication, one way of giving and receiving pleasure.

We bring our bodies to sex. Even more importantly, we bring our minds and emotions. The most important sex organ is not the penis or the clitoris, but the brain. That's where most difficulties with sex start—and where they can be solved. Neither bedroom acrobatics nor 108 titillations from the most exotic sex manual can compensate for severe anxiety, depression, exhaustion, or unwillingness or inability to talk to each other. But the mind, given a chance, can help.

About the time the abdominal incision heals (not many weeks after surgery, barring complications), the doctor will agree that the ostomate can safely participate in the sex act. Before that, of course, caressing, stroking, touching, laughing, cuddling and all the other ways of showing love and caring are fine.

What sometimes happens, the first time, is a scenario like this: Jim, a recent ileostomate, decides that today's the day to make love to his wife for the first time since surgery. If he'll admit it, he's still pretty tired; he doesn't realize how exhausting major abdominal surgery is. Too, he's feeling low — worried about things like money, getting back to work, and problems he can't quite put his finger on. Never mind. He's eager for some good lovemaking. Still, he's a bit anxious. How will it go? What if his appliance slips? What if there's some odor? What if . . .? To calm his fears, he downs a couple of stiff drinks, climbs into bed. Disaster. He can't get an erection. The more he tries, the more frustrated he becomes. Angry and fearful, Jim blames his new ostomy. His wife consoles him—but she wonders too.

It's a classic scene. One surgeon lists four normal (and solvable) problems after surgery: "(a) Failure [of erection or orgasm] because of trying intercourse before strength returns following surgery. (b) Serious anxiety or fear of the ability to perform sexually, the attractiveness of one's altered body, the possibility of odor and the security of the appliance or stoma covering. (c) Depression which many people suffer following any surgery. (d) Excessive medication and/or alcohol."

A different scenario is possible for all the Jims. The next time around, he's a little more rested, he's begun to get some exercise again and to eat well. He's shed a few tears and lost his initial embarrassment. The big difference, though, is that Jim has been talking to his wife, Susan — really talking — and she's been talking too. That old myth of the male as the strong silent type without tears or doubts is just that—a myth. Reality, with men who are not afraid to feel and to talk about what they feel, is better.

Susan has her own worries and resentments. Some fears and angry feelings they can lay to rest. The others they can work on together. Susan admits that a leaky appliance might startle her, but she doesn't see it as a catastrophe. It certainly wouldn't change her love for Jim. After all, they've been through a lot together, including a long siege of illness. Now it's time to delight in his returning health. They've decided that for now they'll just enjoy each other, talking, hugging, touching for the pure pleasure of it without a further goal in mind. Spontaneously, Jim hugs Susan and . . . .

Actually, the first experience with lovemaking after surgery can be great, disappointing, or anything in between. Like one's first experience with sex, it may have more of nerves than of love in it. Yet, if they relax a bit, both partners can enjoy a warm, pleasurable, and rewarding intimacy. Sex, after all, is not performance but sharing.

Probably the most basic factor in sexual intimacy is liking oneself. That feeling of being a worthwhile person — with or without an ostomy—becomes contagious. If we feel good about ourselves, others feel good about us too. If we accept an ostomy, others accept it too. Even in ideal circumstances, it takes time— to become comfortable with a new ostomy, to forget it most of the time, to return to being a person who just happens to have an ostomy, rather than an ostomy with a person attached. Most of us have some doubts about ourselves, even before ostomy surgery. When these doubts are severe enough to interfere with our lives, it's time for professional help.

Jennifer, for instance, was a very attractive single woman, an ileostomate for three years. Her friends were baffled; they introduced pretty, bright, nice Jennifer to young men — but nothing happened. As she was able to laugh about it later, after some therapy, there was a simple explanation. So terrified was she that a date would find out about her ostomy that she froze if he took her hand. If a man put his arm around her, she leaped up with a fragile excuse. She maneuvered her date to the side away from her ostomy. She constantly covered her appliance with her right arm. So frightened was she that a man would find out about her ostomy that she didn't give him a chance to find out about any part of her.

After a few sessions of therapy, Jennifer discovered that she'd used the ostomy as a scapegoat for all the doubts she'd had about herself before surgery. As she became happier about herself, she no longer had to spend all her energy protecting her ostomy — and herself — from discovery. Secure in herself, she was free to learn about other people. (Her last Christmas card mentioned that she and Eric had just celebrated their fifth anniversary; her other big news was the birth of Steven in October.)

Communication is the next critical factor in any sexual meeting. This raises the question: When do I tell him (or her) about my ostomy? "When discovery is imminent" — though a popular answer — may not be the best.

When ostomy surgery happens during a serious ongoing relationship, the partner will probably know all about it from the beginning. But what about a new romance?

As a general rule, the ostomate should tell, at the latest, when it seems possible that intimacy is likely to occur. Before marriage, certainly. Some ostomates feel so much more at ease with their dates *after* they tell them that they make a practice of explaining the ostomy quite early in the friendship.

A simple explanation is sufficient. The UOA booklet *Sex, Courtship and the Single Ostomate* suggests some ways of telling. Basically, an ileostomate, for instance, could say something like this: "I trust you enough to tell you this. I have an ileostomy and I need to wear an appliance." Generally the date looks blank, having no idea what an ileostomy is. The ostomate continues: "I was very sick for a long time. Finally, to save my life, I had serious surgery. I'm perfectly healthy now. But the surgeons made a change in my plumbing—they removed my colon and rectum—now I go to the bathroom differently. I wear a special pouch to collect body waste, so now I can finally do all the things I want to do." If questions follow, the ostomate answers them—clearly, simply, honestly and confidently.

Marlene Vine met her husband in college. "After we had been going together for some time I realized it was time I told him about my ileostomy. I thought, 'Gee, I don't know how he's going to react.' I was so nervous—I had built up such a huge thing in my mind. When I was ready to tell him, he turned to me and said: 'Yes, I know.' That was the last thing I expected to hear!"

At the time, Marlene had worn a rather clumsy appliance, which her boyfriend had felt while embracing her. Bewildered, he had checked with a doctor and then with the library, so that he knew all about the operation before Marlene got around to telling him.

One young woman resolved the "how to tell" dilemma by informing her boyfriend, "I can't go out with you Sunday afternoon. I have a meeting to attend. Would you like to come with me?"—and then taking him to the local UOA meeting!

Most partners who are otherwise right for each other come to accept the ostomy—but it may take time. Mary Ryan admits she was husband-hunting when she met a "very distinguished gentleman" and the friendship thrived—until one evening he told her he had a colostomy: "As I remember, I was very calm and polite, my only feelings at the moment being for him and what an unfortunate situation this must be." She agonized for two days, filled with foreboding and doubts, then visited a nurse's office down the hall from her own office.

"The nurse very briskly and efficiently described a colostomy, even drawing me a picture. She wanted to know my reasons in detail and finished our session with these words of wisdom, 'If this bothers you about an otherwise eligible and fine person, you deserve not even the shadow of a thought from him again.'"

The nurse's insult cleared the air and Mary was able to talk frankly with her man friend instead of working so hard to be consciously kind.

"His insistence that we analyze how I felt about it became masterfully appealing. His honesty, his compassion for me in adjusting to this unknown, and his own basic good sense that a wife-to-be should thoroughly understand, lighted our way. I passed the test with this well-planned tutelage. And, I am proud and happy to say I have the finest, most loving husband in the world."

Although Mary's exploration took time, the resulting understanding became another bond between them.

Ostomy surgery, particularly after long illness, may bring to the surface turbulent, mixed feelings in the partner. Ben Frankel, trying to keep his law practice, two small children and multiple bills in order during his wife's long hospitalization, tells of the painful and ambivalent feelings he faced: "I think underlying it all was the tremendous feeling that I had of anger and resentment that Judy was doing this to me and our family. At the time those feelings started to come up I couldn't really express them, because I knew it was not appropriate for me to feel that way—those were wrong, bad feelings. I had to kind of put them down because you are not allowed to feel angry at your wife because she's sick. I felt angry about the anger, but felt angry anyway! The passage of time helped overcome the feelings of this sort, along with expressing the feelings to yourself first and to other members of your family."

It took a huge argument and a brief separation to clear the air for the Frankels. Until partners can accept these feelings in themselves, communicate them, and begin working together to resolve them, their sex life may suffer. Recognizing that such feelings are normal and common makes them easier to face.

Some partners take longer than Mary and Ben did to accept an ostomy, some less time, and there are a few who never accept it. Either the ostomate or the partner may curtail or even end a sexual relationship, giving the ostomy as the reason; sometimes it's an excuse, a way to camouflage bigger problems. If things don't improve after a reasonable length of time and more information, both partners need to decide if what they share is worth saving. Counseling may help sort out tangled feelings if both want to continue together.

When, as does happen occasionally, a partner does reject an ostomate, the experience can be devastating. Whenever there is rejection by a loved one for *any* reason, it can be devastating. As hard as it is to keep the situation in perspective at the time, it's essential for the ostomate to remember that he or she is still desirable, still basically the same person as before surgery.

Usually though, perhaps after a period of shock and grieving by both partners, a rewarding intimacy can survive—and grow— after ostomy surgery. It's unlikely that such surgery would glue a poor relationship together. But it's even more doubtful if such a change in one's personal plumbing could weaken a sturdy relationship. Many couples have reported a new closeness. Partners find out how much they do mean to each other and rejoice in discovering they both have a growing edge.

A few suggestions about down-to-earth matters may be useful.

Baths and showers are good not only for the stoma area but for sex appeal. Cleanliness is sexy. Even when spontaneity overrides everything else, there's usually time to check that the appliance is fresh, empty, and firmly adhered. Except for the well-regulated colostomate and the ileostomate with a Kock pouch (who may choose a small pad instead of a pouch), ostomates wear appliances during lovemaking.

A slight amount of camouflage may be welcome. Daisy-printed pouches are available, or appliance covers can be purchased or easily stitched at home from a small scrap of fabric. Some ostomates prefer to tuck the appliance under a belt or cummerbund. A number of women, inspired by sexy lingerie catalogs, purchase pretty opaque panties and split the middle of the crotch to about five inches below the waistline, front and back. Cut edges are hemmed and sometimes trimmed with lace or other decoration.

It helps to know—and to assure one's partner—that the stoma won't get hurt during sexplay. Sometimes a partner may wish to see the stoma, sometimes not. A good time is under the shower, or in the bathtub.

Depending on stoma location and appliance, some lovemaking positions may be more comfortable than others. That's where speaking up is important.

Keeping one's sense of humor handy smoothes the way if the unexpected happens. If an appliance slips or a stoma becomes musical at an inappropriate moment, so what? Non-ostomates also pass gas or belch at inappropriate times. A shared laugh, and the world continues to spin.

Something like 50% of all married couples report sex difficulties of one kind or another — and ostomates are not exempt. Many problems can be solved with tenderness, patience, clear talk, and a little more information. Sex counselors can provide the facts; so can reputable sexual manuals. Some doctors are comfortable and knowledgeable about sexual matters; some, unfortunately, are not. ETs, thanks to experience with the problems of many couples, can encourage the new ostomate. They can help make clear, for instance, that the person with a new ostomy may be apathetic about sex for a time after surgery, until the stoma and the new body image are accepted. While the partner needs to be sensitive to this, some initiative may help in conveying the message that this new image is OK.

Although as much as 95% of sex may be mental, that still leaves 5% for plain physical problems. A number of women who have had the rectum removed report painful intercourse for weeks or months after surgery; in most cases, there is a remarkable and satisfying improvement, although it may take time for muscles, nerves, and blood vessels disturbed during surgery to get back to normal. This is a temporary problem; the best remedies are patience, time, gentleness, enough stimulation, and letting one's partner know what feels good.

In the rare case where a woman undergoes extensive surgery of the pelvis with removal of vagina and clitoris as well as of uterus, bowel and bladder, she faces obvious problems. Even in this case, if it's important enough to the individual, plastic surgery may help.

For men, the situation is more complicated. There are four parts to a man's sexual response: erection, ejaculation, orgasm and fertility. No ostomy surgery rules out the possibility of orgasm. Some kinds of surgery, however, may interfere with erection, ejaculation or fertility.

Since the psychological and the physical intertwine in the process of erection, it may take a urologist to decide whether a particular problem results from anxiety or from surgical damage. Most ileostomates find that such problems are temporary. The more radical surgery for cancer causes more damage; some colostomates and urostomates with surgery for cancer report a permanent inability to have an erection, although many others have no problems.

Even when the condition is temporary, the new ostomate may wait months or even years as nerve damage heals before regaining the ability to have an erection. Ed Ward, a past president of UOA and a colostomate, waited 2½ years. His wife, Anne, hadn't met him then but (as she tells it) "... he tells me that regeneration came about gradually. By the time we were married, almost five years following his surgery, he was well within the realm of normal for which we are both grateful. Had he remained impotent, I really don't think it would have made a difference. We love each other dearly and although physical love is important, it is not the only deciding factor in a good marriage. There are many ways to express physical love or to fulfill emotional needs. A tender word, a squeeze of the hand, or a glance across a crowded room are all expressions of love."

A urologist is the one to advise the ostomate about problems with erection. He's also the one who has information about penile implants, one of the newer surgical solutions to physiological problems with erection. So many men with other medical conditions (diabetes is perhaps the most common) cannot achieve an erection that implant surgery is a developing field. Some men have found this mechanical assistance quite satisfactory. Slender rods or inflatable rods are inserted on both sides of the penis; new techniques are appearing all the time. Insurance may or may not cover the relatively expensive operation, which involves two or three days in the hospital.

The grapevine sometimes reports on home remedies for sexual problems—such as a rubber band at the base of the penis for those who can achieve but not maintain an erection. Such self-help can cause serious problems if done incorrectly; a urologist or other knowledgeable health professional can show the safe way to do it.

Probably most people in the world could multiply their pleasure by broadening their sexual horizons—and that includes the ostomate with erection difficulty. The genitals are not the only erogenous zone. The whole body is an immense sensual and sexual network which few of us ever explore fully. All the body can respond to caresses, tenderness and passion. Skin has been called the largest sex organ in the body—and with good reason. Other varieties of sexual experience (manual, oral) can bring deep pleasure. A good sex manual can provide details.

(An ostomy in no way guarantees sterility, so couples who wish to avoid pregnancy need a reliable contraceptive. Women with ileostomies should check that the birth control pill is not passing whole into their appliance. If it is, it's time for another method of contraception.)

In spite of *Playboy* stereotypes, it is wise for everyone—with or without an ostomy — to think of love and sex in the broadest terms, and to be willing to try alternate ways of achieving satisfaction. If it feels good for the two people involved, it is good. There are no standards of comparison. Life is ours to live and enjoy. Sex, always expressed in one way or another, is part of that enjoyment.

"The important thing," adds Dr. Lawrence P. Davis, "is not to make your appliance a chastity belt."

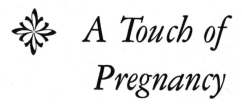 *A Touch of Pregnancy*

To heir is human.
Dolores E. McGuire

"But can I have a baby?"

The young woman queries her doctor, buttonholes the nurse, corners the ET or the ostomy visitor: "Can I have a baby despite my ostomy?"

The answer in almost all cases is a thundering *yes*! Although women with ostomies may choose to skip peanuts or chop suey, there is usually no reason to avoid pregnancy if they want a baby. Women with ostomies are getting pregnant and delivering healthy babies all the time. First babies. Twins. Several babies.

Corrine Barnes, from the Maryland area, claims that when she worked as an ostomy visitor, talking with young women before or soon after ostomy surgery, she heard the question often—and gave the standard answer, that surgery itself does not prevent pregnancy. She goes on to say: "While this is true, it does leave something to be desired as an answer to a very serious question. Now I have a more positive response, and that is that seven years following my ileostomy, I can confirm that pregnancy is very definitely possible. Our first child, Teresa, was born October 11, 1977 at Holy Cross. . . . On November 27, 1978, Teresa's brother Timothy was born."

"Apprehension during pregnancy is certainly not uncommon," writes Janice Hoppes, of Manhattan, Montana, "but don't let an ostomy be your big worry. This, my first pregnancy, proved to be a time of many unfounded fears. With good prenatal care your pregnancy will be as normal as any woman's."

In fact, knowing that women with ostomies can have safe, comfortable, happy pregnancies and deliveries is half the battle. Dr. Albert S. Lyons helped organize one of the first mutual aid groups for ostomates in New York in 1951. He recalls: "When our first ileostomate had a normal delivery, the women in our fledgling ostomy group went flip-flop. Their bellies began expanding. . . . "

Paul Zeit, M.D. draws on years of experience as an obstetrician in a large referral clinic when he reassures doctors and prospective parents: ". . . One learns three very important facts that are not generally understood by most obstetricians, by many surgeons, and by most women who have ostomies of one sort or another. The first fact is that patients with stomas present no different obstetrical problems than patients without stomas. Second, the pregnancy does not create any new surgical problems and it does not alter bowel function in ostomates any more than it does in women with an intact gastrointestinal tract. Third, there are amazingly few mechanical problems with appliances that are brought about by pregnancy."

Doctors tend to advise a wait of a year or two after surgery before conception. Some women, of course, become pregnant before then and generally have uneventful pregnancies, but the body appreciates a chance to heal fully from surgery, to toughen abdominal muscles which may be lazy, and to rebuild nutritional reserves that may have been depleted by bowel disease before surgery. Too, the mother-to-be needs a chance to get accustomed to her stoma before taking on a new baby—plus time to adjust to a new body image before changing it again with pregnancy.

Once a man and woman decide they want a child and are reasonably well prepared for parenthood, a check with the doctor comes next. A phone conversation or visit may be enough to answer questions, to quiet fears. The prospective parents, for instance, learn that even drastic bowel surgery, like removal of one-third to one-half of the small bowel, shouldn't jeopardize the baby's food supply before birth; most food absorption takes place in the first half of the small intestine.

There are a few special cases, of course. A man or woman with ostomy surgery for familial polyps needs to know there is a strong chance that half the children will have polyposis and will require bowel surgery during young adulthood. Women with urinary ostomies must take special precautions against urinary tract infection during pregnancy. Women with ostomies for cancer, especially those who have undergone radiation and/or chemotherapy, need counseling from their doctors.

Finding the right doctor for pregnancy and delivery — before conception, if possible — takes thought. This applies to every woman, with or without an ostomy. Some women already have a doctor in whom they have confidence. Others may follow the recommendation of a friend (possibly of another ostomate friend who has had a baby since surgery), or of their internist or surgeon, or of a teaching hospital in the area. Many doctors have never been present when a woman with an ostomy delivers her child — but this doesn't seem to matter much. As Mary Bir, from Great Lakes, Illinois, warns: "Don't be surprised if your doctor says something like mine did, 'Oh! We don't get too many of your kind.'"

More important than experience with ostomies are the doctor's skill, sensitivity and supportiveness. The doctor who's initially a greenhorn about ostomies can do an expert job, with a little help, perhaps, from the woman's internist or surgeon and from the literature. And many of the general questions which bubble forth from most prospective parents — what about natural childbirth? breastfeeding? fees? — are far more important than the ostomy-related queries.

The woman with an ostomy who becomes pregnant actually enjoys some advantages over her non-ostomate sisters. Writes Mary Bir: "I had a child before and after my surgery. Personally I enjoyed the latter pregnancy much more than my first. One of the many things I did not have to worry about was hemorrhoids and constipation." In fact, since much of the intestine has been removed, there's more room for the growing fetus.

Ostomates are not immune, however, from the common experiences of pregnancy, like a little morning sickness, fatigue alternating with surges of energy, mood swings. And they need to remember the rules which apply to any pregnancy: nutritious diet, regular check-ups, reasonable weight gain.

"There is no reason," states Dr. Zeit, "why she can't carry a pregnancy to term without any more restrictions on her activities than any other woman. . . ."

Ann Wolf confirms Zeit's statement: "My pregnancy was quite uneventful. I continued to work until four weeks before my due date. Then I was so bored at home that I began a new job and even worked the day before the baby was born. We also began packing our belongings because three weeks before my due date we sold our home and had thirty days to move out! We didn't even have a place to move to. So all at once we were packing, looking for a house, and having a baby. Finally we found a house and moved when the baby was only two weeks old." (What does she call an *eventful* pregnancy?)

Some specifics: Many pregnant ostomates find themselves needing more fluids than before. They may notice a change in the consistency of stool, which may become either more liquid or thicker. On some rare occasions, near the end of pregnancy, the uterus will press enough on the intestine to cause a mechanical obstruction; a change of position or, if necessary, a liquid or soft diet for a time solves that problem.

To help prevent or lessen stretch marks, pregnant obstomates can rub a non-oily moisturizer around the incision and all over the belly during that nine months stretch. The doctor may recommend an ointment or lotion for the perineal wound, if any. (Some surgeons, anticipating childbirth, leave the rectum intact during the childbearing years so there is no perineal wound; many obstetricians claim that the perineal scar becomes so elastic during pregnancy that it causes no problems during childbirth.)

Pregnant women with ostomies report remarkably little change in the stoma. Generally it becomes elongated, somewhat oval shaped, and may require a different sized faceplate opening or a reshaped karaya ring. The stoma may increase slightly in diameter temporarily, may protrude a bit more, and, as the blood supply increases to an already well-supplied area, it may bleed slightly. A bigger problem is centering the appliance as baby and belly grow. Ostomates suggest a full length mirror—or a mate's help — and perhaps some paper centering guides for that maneuver. Skin tends to get oilier as pregnancy progresses and some women change appliances more often if adhesion is a problem. Babies also kick around the stoma on occasion; this can cause a little soreness but no real harm.

Women with continent ileostomies have had normal pregnancies and deliveries, without difficulty. Irwin Gelernt, M.D. finds that "the only thing that happens is that the reservoir needs to be emptied more often as the enlarging womb compresses the reservoir. The angle of intubation also changes slightly, but there is no real difficulty with this new angle."

When it's time to go to the hospital, the wise ostomate brings and displays prominently a card with basic information on it: the kind of ostomy, and do's and don'ts — especially no enemas, no laxatives, no rectal temperatures (for those with ileostomies or colostomies). Janice Hoppes expressed her thanks to her thoughtful obstetrician who alerted the small hospital where she planned to deliver her baby so they could brush up on their ileostomy care before she arrived. But not all hospital staffs are so prepared, and the ostomate may need to remind a staff member of basic information about ostomies.

How about delivery? Is a Caesarean section necessary? Dr. Zeit says firmly: "There is no reason for a higher Caesarean section rate in these women than in any other group of women."

Many women, with or without ostomies, wonder if the perineal region will tear during a vaginal delivery. Real problems are rare. Labor and delivery don't harm the stoma or the abdominal incision either.

Some women wear their reusable appliance through labor and delivery while others prefer disposables, bypassing the washing and hanging routine during those hectic first days of motherhood. In those first days there may be a problem maintaining a good seal, since the abdominal contour changes drastically and the skin tends to be flabby for awhile. If leakage occurs, the doctor or ET can suggest remedies.

Janice Hoppes found that she could handle her ostomy care herself after delivery, and was much less embarrassed than she expected to be by such things as her appliance showing while she dressed after showering: "Remember, on an obstetrical floor the only really noticeable objects are the babies in the nursery!

". . . I continued to change my appliance every two days for approximately two weeks following delivery due to my shrinking abdomen to prevent any excoriation. My stoma remains elongated, but the base has returned to its original size."

Concludes Janice: "As a side note on labor and delivery, all new mothers spend time visiting. It was the general consensus that I had probably had the least complicated labor and delivery of any of us. So you can see that an ostomy does not prove to be a barrier during the nine months of pregnancy, nor during the labor and delivery."

CHAPTER 18 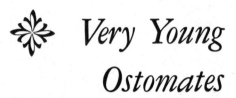 *Very Young Ostomates*

> *Natalie Berenstein of Bexley, Ohio, was six years old when she offered some advice to other very young ostomates: "This is what I would tell another girl or boy about to have an ostomy: Don't be scared about it. Don't get upset. You'll do fine, and you can do anything that you want to do with it!"*

Natalie said it well. Many doctors, ETs and parents of children with stomas would echo her:

CHILDREN WHO NEED OSTOMIES—AND GET THEM — ARE THE LUCKY ONES AND DO WONDERFULLY WELL!

Babies just a few hours old undergo ostomy surgery — and thrive. Preschoolers, given a chance, learn to manage appliances almost as efficiently as their elders — although they may occasionally attach a pouch upside down!

Natalie's surgery was done because of spinal damage present at birth; at the time she advised other young ostomates, she was swimming, riding her bike, playing on the bars of the playgym and working out on a trampoline.

Other very young ostomates may be born with defects in bladder, bowel or anus that require either a permanent or a temporary ostomy. Disease (ulcerative colitis, for instance) or injury may make surgery necessary. If a child suffers repeated kidney infections because of a flaw in the urinary tract, an ostomy may be done to protect the endangered kidneys from further damage. And, as a last resort in cases of incontinence, an ostomy may free a child from endless diapers and plastic pants.

For parents, the news their young child will have an ostomy usually comes as a shattering blow. Shannon Vyff, of Wichita, Kansas, was born without certain important nerves of the descending colon. After trying different treatments, Shannon's pediatric surgeon suggested exploratory surgery to confirm the diagnosis; if the nerves were abnormal, he planned to give Shannon a temporary colostomy. Shannon's mother Janice relives that devastating time: "As the time during the operation dragged on my spirits fell. It took so long, I just knew she had undergone colostomy surgery. I was right. She received her first colostomy, in the descending colon, at four months and one week of age.

"I was so upset. I couldn't stand the idea of my beautiful little daughter being so 'disfigured' in this manner. If my husband had not been there to give me his help and support, I don't know what I might have done. I remained quite bitter about the surgery for a few days.

"Then, at Dr. Mirza's request, a wonderful lady, Rose Randall [an ostomate], came to visit us at the hospital. . . . I decided that if Rose could be so great, an ostomy on Shannon might not be so awful after all.

"And it wasn't! I learned to like Shannon's colostomy, because it made her so comfortable. She immediately started sleeping through the night. Her personality completely changed, and she became an extremely happy baby."

For a time, many urinary diversions were done so a child could be dry. The pendulum has swung to less-permanent solutions, when possible: medicines, bladder massage techniques, self-catheterization (wherein a tube is inserted into the bladder several times a day to drain urine). But sometimes an ostomy is the only answer.

Mrs. Larry Case, of Morgan City, Louisiana, reflects the pain and indecision of the parent forced to make the decision about elective ostomy surgery in a child. Her son Rob had been plagued with bladder and kidney problems since he was five. When the surgery was scheduled, she panicked —as numerous parents do, especially those who have never met and talked with anyone with an ostomy — and cancelled the operation. "At my request his doctor came and my son made the decision that he wanted to be dry. He felt that he would be more like other children that way. I still didn't reschedule the surgery and I had the most terrible week of my life. I suffered for my son's life ahead; the problems he would encounter. Whenever he slept, I cried like it was the end of the world."

Happily, mother and son met a little girl in the x-ray waiting room and discovered that her ostomy pouch didn't show under her dress. But Mrs. Case agonized: "Anyway, I resigned myself to my son's terrible fate. I was assured that in a relatively short time he would be able to care for himself. I didn't have any confidence in this either. I was completely negative. I had no one or nowhere to turn.

"The moral of this story is that all our fears were proved wrong by the one who never had fear. This tiny little boy, who had always been small because he was always so sick, never gave anyone the opportunity to consider him handicapped. He has always been an honor student even with the amount of school he's missed. He is a very good golfer, plays tennis, swims, plays shortstop in Little League and is an outstanding Biddy Basketball player."

Once the go-ahead comes from doctor and parents for ostomy surgery, what then? For the infant in diapers, parents, or the person who usually cares for the child, step in to learn about care. Since the child is already in diapers, there may be no big change in the care—except that the diaper may be a little higher! (The child with an ostomy which produces a liquid stool will need a small appliance to protect the skin from enzymes.)

Pre-schoolers and young school-age children begin to learn

how to care for themselves. Jean Alvers, San Francisco ET, uses a puppet theater to show children what will be happening to them. Play therapy, in which children practice putting appliances on dolls and coping with common problems, helps them vent their own feelings, and increases security in this new situation. *All About Jimmy*, a coloring book available from UOA, helps children understand. Meeting another child with an ostomy can be invaluable for an older child; if that's not possible, talking to an adult with an ostomy can reassure both child and parents.

As children accept glasses or braces, as naturally do they seem to accept ostomies.

Not only parents but older children, grandparents, and babysitters also can learn the basics of caring for the young child's ostomy. This "thing," which seemed at first so horrendous, gradually becomes commonplace and no longer frightening. "Is that all there is to it?" becomes the new question.

Skin care and appliance use require a little special attention with children. Stoma size changes as the child grows and appliances need to be checked for fit frequently. Children may need a few gentle reminders not to skimp on skin care, if they are taking charge of their own ostomy. Basically, as for any ostomate, the appliance-wearing child needs intact skin, an appliance which fits, and a good seal to prevent leakage and promote security.

Many colostomies for young children are temporary, often to bypass the bowel for a few months or years until the child is large enough for corrective surgery. These temporary colostomies are often double-barreled, an arrangement with two stomas next to each other which will eventually be stitched together again. The expert help of an ET can untangle the problems of caring for this more complicated ostomy.

When can a child start caring for an ostomy? In general, children can start assuming responsibility at the toilet training age; if they have ostomy surgery after two or three, they can begin immediately. Emptying the appliance comes first. Then, as the child becomes more mature and dextrous, he or she learns about changing appliances, maintaining the skin, and checking for any problems. Complete independence is the goal. The very young who require assistance receive it, of course, but soon learn to distinguish between a helping hand and having all the care done for them.

As children grow, they strive for adulthood. Dressing themselves, learning to cross the street, and going to school are all steps on this path to gradual independence. So is caring for an ostomy. The parent who continues to care for a child's ostomy past a reasonable age because it's "faster" or "easier" or "better" that way, gives the child the message that he or she "can't do it right." Tying a shoelace may be a challenge when one is five—and so is changing an appliance—but well worth doing.

Parents can help by simplifying procedures and gathering equipment in a place the child can reach. Beyond that, their greatest contribution is in teaching patiently and lovingly—and then stepping back so the child can assume responsibility and the pride that comes with it.

Naomi Remen, M.D., herself an ileostomate and a pediatrician at Stanford University, reminds parents of their crucial role in helping the child with the ostomy: "It is important that the family think of the child as a well child. This is difficult, as often the child has been ill for many months or even years. Now, after his surgery, he is well, and both he and his family must begin to think of him as a competent and total human being. The ostomy and its care should never be used as an excuse for special treatment or privilege. The child should be thought of as a child with, say, glasses or dental braces. These appliances need to be considered in playing sports or traveling, but the consideration should be routine and matter-of-fact."

In some cases, of course, the child has underlying disease, perhaps a spinal defect. But after surgery, the child is *better*. He or she can start meeting the world in ways not possible before the ostomy.

Dr. Remen acknowledges that parents of children with

ostomies may have a hard time making their own adjustments: "They may feel a loss of self-esteem as the parents of a 'defective' child and see the ostomy as a 'flaw' in an otherwise 'perfect' son or daughter. They may feel guilt over what they think is a painful problem they have genetically transmitted to a small child. They may feel resentment towards the child for the worry he has caused and the disruption of family life his illness has represented. They may also resent the financial burden that the illness has imposed on them.

"...Such feelings are common and every attempt must be made to work them through and not communicate them to the child. We learn self-love and self-esteem from our parents. Children are maimed by non-accepting parents and not by a surgical procedure which opens for them the opportunity of a healthy and full life."

The doctor, ETs, other health personnel, and religious counselors or psychotherapists—any may be helpful for parents trying to sort out such feelings.

Dr. Remen suggests open discussion of the ostomy among family and friends of all ages. Concealing the fact may make the child feel ashamed or even maimed. Stories about themselves—how they were sick, how Mommy and Daddy felt, how the doctors helped make them well with the surgery—together with simple, clear explanations of what an ostomy is, are very popular with the younger set.

If the child feels good about himself, a reflection at this young age of the parents' good feelings about the child, he or she is in fine shape to handle any minor storms that arise. Schoolmates and young friends generally accept the situation—often with a little envy! As Rob Case's mother reports: "Other parents have chosen to handle this another way, but being from a small town there was no way for Rob's condition to be a secret. It has worked out beautifully for Rob. All of his friends know, but I don't think they give it a second thought. The mother of one of his classmates told me that her child came home well pleased because 'Rob had a new bag and it sure was pretty.' My six-year-old son says he'd like one also."

It makes sense to inform the school child's teacher and school nurse that the child has an ostomy. The UOA booklet, *My Child Has An Ostomy*, helps explain the facts to a child's school or camp supervisors. An extra appliance set-up can be left at school in case of a leak.

Meeting other children with ostomies, if possible, at ostomy association meetings or through the doctor, ET, or other health personnel (who may know other children with similar surgery), helps immensely, especially for any child who encounters a problem.

Stacy, a very young lady from Evansville, Indiana, sports two ostomies: an ileostomy and ileal conduit. Stacy's mother reports: "Being a very inquisitive child, Stacy has naturally started asking a few questions about her ostomies. We just answer her honestly and simply; she accepts that and is satisfied — just as we, our family and friends have accepted her ostomies, and in fact, count them as blessings. We know that because of her ostomies she is now leading a completely normal and VERY active life."

An ostomy in a child is scarcely a catastrophe. Instead, it is the path to life, in some cases, or to health and dryness.

CHAPTER 19 ✳ *A Word to the Teenagers*

> *Having a colostomy doesn't stop a person from living and enjoying life. I'm not afraid to tell anyone about my ostomy, nor should it be made taboo. I can now eat anything I want. I love salads, fruits, pizzas, etc. I can enjoy everything. I have a girlfriend, in fact more than one.*
> Mark Singer

Mark Singer, of Metro Maryland Youth Ostomy Association, didn't always accept his ostomy so happily. When doctors told him they planned a colostomy for his Crohn's disease, Mark balked: "I thought it was the worst thing that could happen to anyone. When I heard the word and the way it was put to me I wanted to die."

Jim Clark went a little further. He accepted surgery (he thought) and then tried to check out of the hospital the night before his operation was scheduled: "I was so scared. . . . So they notified security and security picked me up at the gate. I was kind of obvious, because I was the only one wearing a nightgown!" Even after he was returned to his room, Jim barricaded the door.

What made the difference for both Mark and Jim was another ostomate. Mark's mother called Metro Maryland Ostomy

Association; president Horace Saunders came and visited every day before surgery and every day afterwards. For Jim, it was an ostomate whom the hospital contacted after Jim's attempted escape. The ostomate showed up right before Jim's surgery: "I always thought that ostomates were green people who were really wild, but he was a normal-looking person and he came to see me at four o'clock in the morning to wish me good luck. That's all I needed. . . ."

Many young people have ostomies. Some have had them for a long time, maybe even since they were babies. Some choose an ostomy as they grow up after struggling for years with constant wetness and diapers for a birth defect or urinary tract problem that couldn't be corrected any other way. A few teenagers have ostomies after an accident in which their bowel or urinary tract is injured. But most young people who undergo ostomy surgery have ulcerative colitis or another bowel disease.

When you've been sick for a long time with a bowel disease, you may be so anxious to get rid of the pain and misery that you really don't care much how it happens. But an *ostomy*? Having to wear a "bag" everywhere? That sounds even worse than the disease. Especially when you're weak and sick, that may seem like the last straw.

That's how it seemed to Naomi Remen. She had an ileostomy at 17 for ulcerative colitis, although she couldn't stand even the thought of an ostomy and decided not to learn how to put on an appliance. Secretly, she plotted to kill herself upon leaving the hospital. But after she went home, she received a phone call from a female member of the local ostomy association. Naomi refused to see her, but the persistent woman said she would come anyway. One look at a beautiful woman in a tight skirt — and Naomi decided life might be worth living after all. (She eventually became a pediatrician, and frequently writes articles about ostomies and young people.)

There *are* special problems for teenagers. You're trying to find out just who you are. You want to be yourself, an individual, but not too different from everyone else. It's not easy to think of yourself as a normal, healthy person when you're sick all the time. An ostomy can make you a healthy person again, but it's hard—at first — to keep from feeling really different from everyone else. When you first have an ostomy, it's difficult to convince yourself that other people aren't aware of it, unless you tell them. But once you've learned the basics of caring for an ostomy, other people don't need to know. An ostomy is much easier to hide than acne or a pudgy middle.

One of the big hassles for a lot of young people is becoming independent. Accepting the authority of doctors and parents to make decisions about *you* (e.g., you need an ostomy) can raise the rebel in any teenager. When you've been sick a long time, you may find it hard to get parents to accept the fact that you're healthy now and can start having more say in your life. On the other hand, when you've been used to some special attention and pleasant coddling, you may not feel like giving it up. Some days all teenagers wish they could be young children again, with parents caring for their every need. Other days they'd like to be completely grown up and on their own with no one telling them what to do. This emotional teeter-tottering is just part of growing up—although that doesn't make it any easier to accept.

Often it's hard to understand how parents feel, especially when you have your hands full already coping with your own problems —one of which may be parents! Some parents feel guilty because you've been sick; they may wonder if they might have prevented it by doing something differently. Since a lot of parents are reluctant to see their children grow up and away from them, they may want to baby you, either during illness or after an ostomy. Some parents have difficulty accepting any disease or problem in their "perfect" children. Other parents may harbor resentments about the emotional and financial drains the illness has made on them; these are normal feelings, no matter how much parents love a child, but since most parents would feel guilty about expressing them directly, the resentment crops up in strange places where it can really hurt.

Sometimes it's *really* hard to decipher the meaning behind what a parent says. One participant at a Youth Rap Session at the 1974 UOA Conference faced such a parent problem: "I went out on a date with a young man and when I came back my father said: 'Did you have a good time?' And I said: 'Yes, blah, blah, blah—this is where we went, this is what we did.' My father said: 'Too bad he can't afford the medical bills, isn't it.'

"Right after your surgery, you have this new little thing there on your side, and you are wondering how people are going to accept you; what you are going to do. You go out on a date and you come back and your dad says that, it's like putting you back about six months."

As devastating as the father's comment was — and many a parent has made some similar statement to a teenager, ostomate or not—one of the subtler messages behind the words actually may be something like this: "I, your father, *can* pay your medical bills. I may not be as young and handsome as this kid, but I'm still your dad and I'll take care of you. . . ." Growing up means becoming independent of parents and that rarely happens smoothly. There are bumps and curves along the way, for all teenagers, all parents.

Especially after a long illness, you may feel like Rip Van Winkle re-entering the world. Even if you participated in school and activities during the illness before an ostomy, so much of your energy was tied up with being sick, that it was kind of a half-hearted participation. Young people are not known for their patience, and this period of catching up—with school, with social life, with thinking about a career—isn't easy. One good friend can help a lot—or a school counselor or a favorite teacher. There are a lot of people willing to help.

Just about every teenager experiences rejection by someone, at some time, for some reason. A few people may not accept you because of the ostomy, usually because it's something so new to them. As Mark Singer says: "My friends couldn't say ileitis or colitis, let alone know what it was like. But today they are getting an education because I'm speaking out and making others aware of the various aspects of ostomies."

Not everyone handles the situation that way. Some young adults prefer not to tell others about the ostomy. That's one nice thing about an ostomy: because it's hidden, you can tell other people or not.

If any big problem arises—and stays big for quite awhile—it's worth getting help. A teacher, or school counselor, or doctor, or ET may be able to help or may be able to suggest someone else who can help. Getting help for a big problem doesn't mean you've failed; it means instead that you are mature enough to know and use other resources.

Some of the questions that young ostomates ask are ones older ostomates ask too: How do I tell people? What about dates? What about sports? How about getting a job? Other chapters in this book talk about those subjects.

But there are some questions specific to teenagers. The United Ostomy Association is beginning to recognize the special needs and questions of young people. Youth groups within chapters are springing up all over the U.S. so that young ostomates can help each other with practical, personal information—and so they can have fun in the process. In youth groups, teenagers, and those a little younger and a little older, meet each other and make new friends, have a chance to think and talk about these new changes in their bodies, exchange ways of coping with them, and learn about the latest in appliances. Picnics, dances, other social events may be on the agenda. One of the most important jobs of members is contacting other young people about to have ostomy surgery or who have just had it.

United Ostomy Association, Inc. (2001 West Beverly Boulevard, Los Angeles, California, 90057) is the source to contact to find a chapter in your area. If there isn't a youth group within the chapter, it may be possible to find an ostomate pen-pal. Or the regular UOA chapter may work out well for you.

Nobody ever said it was easy to be a teenager.

When you're a teenager, the good times are not just good — they're incredible. But the bad times are so bleak that it's hard to believe there will ever be a good moment again. Adults may say, "Oh, it's going to get better. Stop mooning around and feeling sorry for yourself" — but that doesn't help at all.

All young people — with or without ostomies — face many of the same doubts, ask the same questions. Most are searching for independence; most are trying to live with bodies that are changing drastically and are frequently unpredictable (except that the big pimple *always* shows up on the night of the important date!). Most teenagers crave acceptance by other teenagers — and aren't always sure that they are accepted. Most wonder what they will do with their lives. Most are experiencing new feelings and sensations and relationships—and aren't too sure about any of it yet.

On the other hand, after an ostomy they may share the basic good health and high spirits common to young people. And they have a great capacity to make changes — to adapt to this slight change in the plumbing.

Talking with a friend—sharing good times and bad—seems to be one of the best ways to survive the teenage years. And when the questions and doubts are about an ostomy, the United Ostomy Association proves a faithful friend. As Marlene Vine puts it, it's "a one-to-one thing where someone has helped you, and you, in turn, help someone else."

CHAPTER 20   ❧   *Check-ups and Follow-ups*

Being discharged from the hospital didn't mean quite as much freedom as I'd hoped; the doctor said to come back in two days. . . .

"Isn't it about time for your next appointment with the doctor?" my daughter asks.

"Maybe so. I'd better check." A foolish answer. I know the date better than my own birthday.

"How are you feeling?" she continues.

"Oh, fine." That's not quite true, either. Secretly I've written down a list of ten mysterious and probably dangerous symptoms to ask him about. And I'm working on number eleven.

We both know that somehow, just before a check-up, my medical imagination seems to go on a rampage. The tiniest symptom automatically means disaster, and I can see my entire intestinal tract coming apart as I wait.

In most cases, the actual check-up turns out to be a helpful, even comforting visit with a doctor I know and like. If there's a problem, it often gets a name. That makes it more manageable, and together we can search for a solution. After the appointment,

I laugh at all that stupid, needless worry. I won't do that again. At least not until the next check-up....

For our friends who've had ileostomies to cure ulcerative colitis, surgery usually means the end of frequent and frustrating medical check-ups. After all, a non-existent colon cannot become inflamed.

For most of the rest of us — whether the problem is Crohn's disease, cancer, or something else—regular check-ups are now a part of the game, although the time between medical appointments soon stretches. Every other day becomes once a week, then once a month, three months, six months, a year. If surgery followed the discovery of cancer, touching base regularly usually continues for the rest of one's life.

Much research, time and money has gone into the quest for an easy and sure test to identify cancer cells anywhere in the body, as accurately as a Geiger counter finds certain metals. Such a test would simplify early detection and thus multiply cures. Preliminary experiments with certain tests (the CEA or Carcino-embryonic Antigen blood test, for instance) hold promise for the future but still need to be perfected.

Until such a magic tool is found, doctors vary in the checks they make and the tests they order. Along with my list of ten scary questions (and a pad and pen for jotting down answers), I soon learned to take along a spare appliance in case the doctor wanted to examine my stoma. At least at first, stoma and perineal wound (if there is one) are frequently inspected. There are also a variety of blood and urine tests. Weight is usually a routine check, along with periodic chest x-rays. Those who have urostomies may have IVPs (kidney x-rays) as part of their ritual. At any sign of trouble, still more sophisticated tests—bone scans, liver scans, and ultrasound x-rays for instance—may be ordered.

It's doubtful that anyone will ever become addicted to barium enemas and the x-rays which accompany them. Still, for many colostomates (ileostomates *never* have barium enemas), they are a necessary nuisance. In some ways, the procedure is not as uncomfortable after a colostomy as it was before.

Some x-ray staffs understand colostomies; many do not. The ostomate may need to use a little polite, informed assertiveness. For instance, the extended diet preparation and harsh laxatives usually ordered before rectal barium enemas may be overkill for the colostomates. Some x-ray staffs accept irrigation just before a barium enema as an adequate substitute for the laxatives. For those who don't irrigate, a gentler laxative than those prescribed for non-ostomates hopefully can be agreed upon.

Many ostomates, whether they irrigate or not, take along an irrigation cone to be slipped on the tube carrying the barium in lieu of the longer standard catheters. Instead of a cone, a soft Foley catheter can be used (this has an inflatable balloon on it so that the barium stays inside the stoma).

Whether a cone or Foley is used, it should be lubricated with surgical jelly and inserted gently but firmly into the stoma, preferably *by the ostomate*. To keep the barium in, it is necessary to hold the cone firmly in place until the test is over. An adhesive-type disposable irrigating sleeve may help control the barium, which wants to spurt all over the room the second the cone is removed.

Although some of the barium will splash out immediately, some will remain. Even when it is possible to irrigate immediately afterward in a nearby bathroom, the ostomate should wear an appliance home. More than one ostomate, released from x-ray with a gut still partly full of barium and no appliance, has whitewashed his clothes and painted a pinkish white stripe from front door to bathroom.

The opposite problem which can arise with barium is severe constipation. As the water which keeps the barium in suspension is absorbed by the colon, the insoluble barium hardens quickly in the intestine. The colostomate should irrigate as soon as possible afterward, or take an approved laxative. Abundant fluids and food (especially items with a good percentage of fiber) also help prevent barium blockage.

During the last few years, many doctors have begun to substitute colonoscopy through the stoma for the barium enema.

After the bowel is emptied, with the same preparation as for the barium enema, the doctor inspects the colon through the flexible lighted tube; pieces of tissue for biopsy can be removed, if necessary. Some medicine to relax the ostomate is given before the procedure.

As surgical techniques have improved, the need to revise stomas has decreased. Most problems—if any—develop during the first year. Many can be solved without surgery. Occasionally, scar tissue causes blockage and must be removed. If a stoma retracts (draws in) or prolapses (protrudes) farther than it should, causing management problems, surgical correction may be necessary. Sometimes an ostomate can get a hernia near the stoma. In most cases, the problem is not severe enough to require surgery.

For people with a temporary ostomy, it sometimes takes many check-ups before it's time to reconnect the intestine (and do away with the stoma). Months or even years may pass before everything is right for the switch back. The reasons for such procedures are so varied that there can be no general rules. In many cases, although the surgery is major, reconnection is easier than the operation which created the temporary colostomy or ileostomy. For one thing, the individual is apt to be in far better health. For another, there are few surprises when one knows what to expect. Once in awhile, there's a surprising twinge of doubt: the ostomy's working so well—why not just leave it alone!

On any trip to the hospital (whether to have a stoma revised, a baby, or an ingrown toenail removed), the person with an ostomy may need to help educate hospital staff, especially on non-surgical floors where ostomates may be rare birds. The ostomate can bring along two cards with basic information on them, one to give to the admitting nurse so that facts can be recorded on the Nursing Kardex (the file where basic information about the patient is written), the other to display prominently on the bedside table. As an example, an ileostomate who has had her rectum removed might include this information: *ATTENTION: Patient has an ileostomy. Do not take rectal temperature. Do not give enemas. Do not give laxatives. Do not irrigate ileostomy. Do not remove appliance from abdomen.* Even with these cards, the ostomate may have to speak up—loudly—if a nurse approaches with a rectal thermometer.

Since not all hospitals know that Joe Blow's Velvet Touch Pouches are the best in the world, experienced ostomates learn to bring their own appliances and supplies, including an irrigation set and disposable irrigation sleeves if used, and, for the sake of staff and roommates, a supply of a pouch deodorant or satisfactory room deodorizer. An IV pole can hold the irrigation bag, but is too high; a wire coat hanger bent so there is a strong hook at each end solves the problem. Many colostomates choose to forget irrigating if they're bed-bound. Once they're up and around again, they can get back on schedule with little trouble. In the meantime, lightweight disposable and drainable pouches allow them freedom to concentrate on getting well.

When ostomy surgery follows the discovery of cancer, the doctor may recommend radiation and/or chemotherapy, which may increase the effectiveness of the surgery. Radiation can further shrink tumors and destroy any cancer cells still lurking in the immediate area. Chemotherapy uses powerful drugs to combat stray cancer cells anywhere in the body. Immune therapy, often classified as a form of chemotherapy, stimulates the body's own defense system so it will recognize and destroy cancer cells wherever they are.

Both chemotherapy and radiation are strong medicine, offering many potential benefits and some potentially unpleasant side effects.

Radiation, which may be done before or after surgery, involves a carefully worked out series of treatments. The radiation therapist aims the powerful beam at the cancer site, where it will do the most good, and carefully shields other areas so the tissues will not be damaged. The treatments are not painful, but they can cause skin problems (usually temporary), nausea and vomiting (often helped by medication), and other side effects.

Chemotherapy has brought about dramatic improvements and

cures with some kinds of cancer. In others, it is still at the experimental stage. Most of the drugs used work best on cells which divide quickly. To date, they are less effective with slower growing tumors (which include many colo-rectal cancers). The fast growing cells which chemotherapy drugs attack include not only cancer cells but also hair cells and the cells lining the digestive tract, leading to such side effects as hair loss, nausea and vomiting. Medication and conscientious attention to basic nutrition can help with nausea, vomiting and other digestive problems. Relatively new techniques such as applying ice to the scalp or a tourniquet around the hair line often prevent hair loss.

Chemicals are given by mouth, by injection into muscle or vein, or by other routes. Schedules vary greatly; some are started on an in-patient basis and then continued as out-patient treatment. Since chemotherapeutic agents are extraordinarily powerful, personnel administering them must use all their knowledge and ingenuity to protect or "rescue" non-cancerous cells during treatment. In every case, doctors and patients must weigh possible benefits against probable problems. As with any other treatment, attitudes are important. Emotional support, medication to offset side effects, and interesting diversions are all part of the program. With both radiation and chemotherapy, tempting and nutritious food is an essential ally.

The techniques for using these powerful tools, their possible benefits, and their side effects (along with ways to prevent them) are all part of complicated and ever-expanding field. Specific information is best obtained from the specialists — oncologists and radiotherapists—by asking as many questions as necessary to feel comfortable with the choice, and possibly requesting a second opinion.

ETs suggest regular appointments during the first year and recommend checking in once in a while after that. There may be a new appliance which will solve a lot of problems; weight gains may have changed the kind or size of appliance needed. Often, little tiny problems never get a chance to grow large if they're spotted when they're small.

In a novel, *To Build A Ship*, Don Berry has something to say about survival: "Man is by nature a victim. But when he knows he can survive anything—he rebels, and is no longer a victim. He feels the power of his own surviving in his belly and it makes him wake up in the middle of the night and turn under his blankets with a secret smile. For the first time he realizes there is more to living than merely submitting. . . ."

Check-ups are one of the resources that help us feel the power of our own surviving, and turn under our blankets with a secret smile. . . .

CHAPTER 21 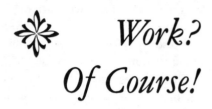 *Work?*
Of Course!

> *Work — keep everlastingly at it, for it is the*
> *darlingest gift of the gods.*
> Mark Twain

There are times—like the Monday morning commute rush—
when our zeal for work may not match Twain's. But satisfying
work is a blessing (and pays the bills), and an ostomy seldom
prevents an individual from finding or keeping a job.

If the word of thousands of doctors, stenographers, truck
drivers, housewives, salespeople, nurses, teachers, bricklayers,
professional athletes, musicians, mailmen, volunteers, scientists,
plumbers, mechanics, policemen, and other ostomates means
anything, people with ostomies do just about everything—and
do it well. Every time someone suggests an occupation for which
an ostomate is unfitted, someone else has on the tip of the tongue
the account of an ostomate in that job. Ostomates used to take it
as gospel that they could be anything—except belly dancers or
professional football players. Then a belly dancer and a professional football player turned up with ostomies.

It's a third-hand tale, but one ostomate insists that a San

Francisco Bay Area doctor has a patient who worked in a rodeo; after surgery, the doctor told the new ostomate he could return to his job. "Later he found out the patient rides Brahma bulls and so the doctor asked the man if it didn't create a problem. The patient said: 'Yeah, I lost my bag but I didn't mind, the bull didn't mind, and I won anyway!'"

As Ed Gambrell, a past president of UOA, says flatly: ". . . an ostomy is not an illness. It is the fully manageable result of a procedure to *cure* an illness or to *remedy* a disorder."

Richard Daniels, a food chemist who has lived and worked with an ileostomy for over a quarter of a century, suggests four basic questions for the ostomate thinking of a job:

1. Am I physically able to do the job?

2. Will my employer take me back? (Or will this employer hire me?)

3. Will I be accepted by my fellow employees?

4. Will my changed bathroom habits cause any problems?

Am I physically able to do the job? Until the new ostomate recovers from surgery and learns to live comfortably with the ostomy, the thought of lifting anything heavier than a toothbrush may be overwhelming. Even after full recovery from surgery, people have different levels of energy and strength to balance against the physical demands of a particular job. Most of the time, if the person with the ostomy really wants *that* job, there is a way to make it possible.

The ostomate thinking about a job requiring very heavy lifting, for instance, may find it sufficient to wear a sturdy support garment and to review the best ways to lift heavy objects—or he may want to set his sights on a job without such heavy lifting. In a very hot job, like on the fire line of an aluminum plant, the ostomate may need to consume Gatorade® by the gallon to ward off dehydration. A comfortable cushion can ease the twinges of a still tender perineal wound for an ostomate who drives a bus.

Will my employer take me back? Or will this employer hire me? These questions don't arise at all for the self-employed. The lawyer, the housewife, the artist, the store owner can return to the job without breaking step. And many ostomates, their surgery time covered by accumulated sick leave, rejoin their company without a ripple of a problem.

Others may find a few obstacles on the path. If the employer has an opening, and if the ostomate has the experience, ability and desire to fill that opening, the employer still can have some reasonable questions: What is the past work and absenteeism record? What is the prognosis for this person after this kind of surgery? Is this employment going to create any special problems for me, the employer?

A personal physician or the medical adviser of the local UOA chapter can smooth the way. If absenteeism before surgery was a problem — very common if chronic bowel disease led to the ostomy—the doctor can reassure the employer: the ostomy should decrease the absences. Questions about prognosis too can be answered in a phone call or letter from the physician.

Some employers balk at hiring or rehiring an ostomate because they don't know much about ostomies and it's easier just to say "no." What ostomates take for granted is completely foreign to some employers who may not even know what an ostomy *is*, let alone that a person can live a normal, comfortable, productive life with one. Some basic information and gentle assertiveness by both ostomate and physician can topple old prejudices and can answer specific questions about such matters as company insurance, physical ability, worker's compensation. After all, as Ed Gambrell points out, "an ostomate's employability should be given thoughtful and fair consideration, not just on behalf of the ostomate who may already be employed or who is looking for a job, but also in the interest of the employer who seeks to hire and retain good employees."

Will I be accepted by my fellow employees? *If the ostomate accepts the ostomy, others will too.* Doing the job and treating others with consideration (leaving the bathroom clean and odor-free, for instance) are essential. Whether or not to tell fellow employees about an ostomy is a personal choice; since the ostomy is invisible under work clothes, no one will know unless the ostomate wishes to tell. Many ostomates hesitate to tell others until they are well established in a job, and then tell one or two friends. Others share their experiences more readily.

Will my changed bathroom habits cause any problems? It is more comfortable to have access to a convenient bathroom. If appliances need frequent drainage or expulsion of air, ostomate and supervisor may need to arrange for a desk closer to the bathroom or perhaps for shorter, more frequent "coffee breaks."

Many people—students, women entering the job market after staying home with a family—apply for their first paid job after an ostomy. A shaky job market and lack of employment experience cause far more problems than the ostomy. School counselors, Department of Employment counselors, classes on getting a job —all can help.

Other people with ostomies change jobs after surgery. Some choose new careers in the health field—sometimes as doctors or nurses or enterostomal therapists—as a direct result of their own experiences. Many reassess their priorities after surgery and decide to pursue a career they always wanted to follow but, for one reason or another, never did. Some find that the stress level of the pre-surgery job is unacceptable and find a job where there is less, or different, stress. Some, freed for the first time in years from chronic bowel disease, explore the many new avenues open to them.

And some people just want a change, like Jim Holladay who turned from contracting to serious carpentry after his colostomy —at age 88!

For the person with an ostomy who cannot, for any good reason, return to a former occupation, sometimes the local office of the state bureau of vocational rehabilitation can finance job re-training if the doctor recommends it. It's worth considering, if there's a problem.

One big question for job-seeking ostomates is "How much do I tell the Personnel Office?" David Rightman of the Los Angeles Department of Employment wishes that more ostomates would pioneer, volunteering full information to their prospective employers. That way, he contends, more employers would know about the excellent ostomate employees they have already and would be more willing to hire other ostomates.

But, when the current employment situation is tight, many ostomates prefer to downplay the ostomy, perhaps informing the employer *after* a period of satisfactory employment. This does not mean lying or falsifying answers, of course. But as Ed Claitman, from Pittsburgh, counsels: "One question that continually comes up from many, many people applying for employment with corporations is under the heading of 'Do you have a physical handicap?' We consistently recommend that you answer 'NO,' as we do not consider an ostomy a handicap. If there is a question about surgery, within a specific time limit, obviously you must honestly answer that question. It boils down to the fact that unless the question is very, very specific, where to AVOID mentioning an ostomy is a false statement, then do nothing to bring it out."

When Mary St. John started looking for a job in the 1960s, she had a new ileostomy after five months of hospitalization for ulcerative colitis: "It was at that point that I first came up against the cruel, hard world. As far as I was concerned, I felt I was perfectly healthy and normal and in much better shape than many of my peers. But with this terrible medical history, I found that most companies were a little reluctant — and that is an understatement!—to have anything to do with an ostomate. I had a lot of doors slammed in my face and I was pretty unhappy about it. One of the things I did was apply at many of the companies that are government contractors, and they usually require security clearance. You have to go through this very involved rigamarole of filling out complicated forms, and there is always a little block about medical history. I was so candid and honest about this I think, perhaps, I was frightening some people. We are all very comfortable and relaxed about ostomy surgery, but for people who are not familiar with this sort of thing it is a shock, and they are sometimes taken up short by it.

"I finally made up a little plan. I don't like to think of this as dishonest. I'd like to think it is one of those sins of omission. When I would come to the little spot in the application which said, 'Have you ever had serious illness or surgery?' I would say, 'Yes, in 1964 I had an intestinal infection. The condition was surgically cured by removal of the infected section of the intestine.' And that was that. I was finally employed by a very well-known company which I stayed with for about two and a half years. Two months ago, I left it and went to work for my present employer. He knew about my ileostomy, but I had to fill out the form and take a physical. So I hied myself off to the handy dandy little company physician and went through the whole chest thumping thing. He looked at my form and said, 'Well, now Miss St. John, I see you've had some surgery. How is your colitis?'

"'Just fine, it never bothers me. I no longer have a colon, so I don't have much trouble with colitis,' and that was the end of that!"

Most ostomates who want a job and are otherwise qualified get a job eventually, although there may be missteps along the way— which one can laugh at, *later.* Don Binder, Executive Director of UOA and a commercial artist, was refused when he applied for his first job after surgery: ". . . I didn't qualify for the company's insurance program. I offered to waive the insurance but that wasn't acceptable. The disconcerting part was that the examining physician kept calling my ileostomy a colostomy. I couldn't understand how a doctor could confuse the two when I knew well the difference."

Now that there are more ostomates around, with more collective clout in the job market, some of the thornier issues like insurance and worker's compensation are being resolved. The more personal elements of job-seeking and keeping — liking oneself, ostomy and all, and communicating that good self-image to employer and other employees — come easily to some ostomates, less easily to others. Talking to ostomates with jobs can help. Concentrating on the job to be done rather than on one's self can carry one smoothly through the job application process and those first few days of work.

What if the person with an ostomy applies for a specific opening for which he or she is well qualified, takes care with the job interview (comes on time, neatly dressed and so on), answers satisfactorily any questions about past absenteeism, current prognosis, physical ability, insurance, worker's compensation (with the help of the personal physician or the medical advisor of the local UOA chapter, if necessary)—and still doesn't get the job? What then?

The UOA formed a national committee to investigate problems related to the employment of ostomates—and disbanded it a few years later because there wasn't enough for it to do. Job discrimination simply because of an ostomy is rare. But UOA remains a resource, if there is evidence of such discrimination. The state department of employment is a possibility. If a cancer diagnosis is the stumbling block, the Cancer Society (American or Canadian) may be able to help.

The larger picture — showing employers everywhere that an ostomy is no bar to employment — gets better all the time. TV programs, newspaper stories, service club programs all spread the word. But individual ostomates working well in individual jobs spread the word most effectively.

When Linda Schwartz graduated from the University of Southern California School of Pharmacy, she was hired as one of the full-time pharmacists—at the hospital where she had become an ileostomate at the age of six.

Or there's Horace Saunders, the force behind the UOA national Youth Movement, who continues to work at his chosen profession as a custom tailor with a clientele that includes movie stars and senators.

Or Marilou Tinay who returned to her job as an airline

stewardess after a complete jejunostomy (leaving only 13 inches of small intestine) for Crohn's disease—and runs an ostomy supply store in her "spare" time.

Or there's. . . .

CHAPTER 22 ❋ *Swimming,*
Skiing and Other
Diversions

Although I'll never be quite as eager a sports person as my friend
Carol Norris, I can't blame my inertia on my ostomy. Carol, on
the other hand, is a runner, thanks to her ileostomy. Before that
happened, she says, she was a Florida-grown indoor type who
preferred curling up with a book to running. . . .

The way Carol tells it, "After my ulcerative colitis ileostomy at
27, I hiked, but preferable downhill, and without a back-pack. At
38 I began jogging, and at 40 I'd reached three miles, three times
a week. That is the turning point for easily doubling distances.
My husband shamed me by reaching marathon-running in his
first six months, while I kept coming in last at club races of 2-5
miles. When a boy of 4 and woman of 70 ran in our local
marathon, I decided to train harder. Now I've run two
half-marathons (13.1 miles each) and hope someday to better that
distance."

Since people with ostomies are people first, their reasons for
choosing any physical activity are basically those of anyone else: to

feel good, to be healthy, and to enjoy the activity. As Carol pinpoints it, "How I regret the lazy years when I did no jogging, when I had to watch my diet, enlarge my clothes, and gasp on one flight of stairs. . . . Let your body assert itself and find health. Hit the road, sisters!"

An ostomy is certainly no hindrance to sports of all kinds — running, jogging, swimming, sailing, skiing, bowling, golf, bicycling and tennis, to name a few. Babe Didrickson Zaharias won the U.S. Women's Open Golf Championship in 1954, *after* her colostomy for cancer in 1953. People with ostomies participate as gymnasts, fencers, football players, sky-divers, skin divers, and hockey players. Name the sport and there are ostomates involved, playing hard, with no limit on their enjoyment.

Even the simplest exercise does wonders for getting and keeping abdominal muscles firm, and appetite and digestive tract in good order. Swimming and walking are among the best. In the months just after surgery, this may mean sauntering instead of a twelve-mile hike, or only a lap or two of a swimming pool instead of twenty (time enough later for the Mark Spitz act). Whatever kind it is, activity speeds healing.

Before surgery, I'd enjoyed the pool in the courtyard almost daily, so I was eager to return to swimming, especially during the hot August days. After checking with my doctor, I cautiously and rather self-consciously edged down the pool steps, picking a time when the pool was almost deserted. My legs had as much power as two soggy strands of spaghetti — they wouldn't kick. Besides, I was worrying about my appliance leaking or showing. Even so, the water felt wonderful, lapping my body, soothing yet invigorating. Maybe I was getting well — except for those lazy legs.

A few hints before I tried the pool could have increased my confidence — and pleasure. If I'd known abdominal muscles (which have a lot to do with controlling leg movements) almost always take time to regain their tone after major surgery, I'd have been less upset by temporarily wilted legs. And if I'd tried reading in the bathtub for an hour or so, complete with appliance and bathing suit, before trying the pool, I wouldn't have worried about appliance security.

There are other common sense tips for swimmers. If a belt is used, it should be rubber or nylon, perhaps worn a little more snugly than usual; elastic belts stretch when wet. Waterproof tape, put on dry skin in picture frame fashion around the outer edges of the faceplate, will hold most appliances securely. Although skin barriers are not generally exposed to water, karaya is water soluble. To be completely safe, other choices may be better for swimming. A thin panty girdle or jockey-type shorts may be worn under a swimsuit or men's swimming briefs. Style depends not only on stoma location but on personal preference— and current fashion. There are bikini wearers among ostomates, but many feel more comfortable with one-piece suits (albeit with plunging necklines), and some like suits with a skirt, or belted shift styles.

Most new ostomates need to take it easy at first. There is the recent surgery to recover from, one day at a time. Many, too, are free for the first time in years from an illness which kept them sedentary and thus out of condition.

Even those in superb condition before surgery, like Otto Graham, captain, U.S. Coast Guard Academy, and former professional football star with the Cleveland Browns, may find it necessary to go slow at first. Graham discovered that being forced to try a slower pace had a real, if unexpected, advantage. An active tennis player and golfer before surgery, he believes his games are "...as good if not better than they were before my operation.

"In golf, I was so weak at first I had to swing very slowly and let the club do the work. As everyone knows, this is the best way to swing a golf club; swing easy and let the club do the work. And this has carried over, even though I have regained my strength."

Teenage hockey player Richard Alperin, of Holbrook, Massachusetts, rebelled at taking it easy at first and started playing ice hockey two short months after his continent ileostomy. This didn't give his new internal pouch enough time to heal securely. But five months after a second surgery, Richard was back on the ice, this time with no ill effects. He has since gotten his high school diploma and started working: "I get a lot of exercise and wouldn't consider working at a job which wasn't physical....I'm a very active person and enjoy getting completely exhausted."

Evan Deutsch, of Southfield, Michigan, began running marathons after ostomy surgery. After gaining 50 pounds in the two months following his ileostomy, he had decided the most enjoyable way to stay lean—was to run.

Aside from the pleasure of participating, and the good things physical activity does for one's general health, ostomates know that sports heal mind as well as body. Exercise remains one of the best ways around for dealing with anger, depression, worry, and increased stress, problems that frequently show up as disease in the body. While there are other elements to bowel disease and cancer, many doctors feel that the body's reaction to emotional stress remains important. Physical activity, by providing an outlet for stress, is one of the best medicines available.

Runner Michael Komlos sets himself a goal of 3000 miles a year. "I remember when I first started to run I was really out of breath. I came back home after running two miles and laid down on the kitchen floor. I thought I was going to die. But after a short rest, I went right back outside and started to run again."

Michael claims that he runs for health, but "just as importantly, I run for my spiritual and mental well being."

"I can really be alone with my thoughts when I'm running. It's just a total release."

Ostomates also point to the confidence they get with sports. Self-image problems (often enormous right after the surgery) recede as ostomates are able to say to themselves, "Look what I can do!"

Lori Musser, a gymnast from Tucson, Arizona, had her ileostomy when she was 11, after a two-year bout with colitis. As she tells it, "I started my freshman year in high school on the tennis team. I wasn't much of a tennis player, but with a lot of practice, I got to where I could get the ball over the net (part of the time!). I was at the bottom of the ladder most of the time, it was something I was accustomed to because, before my surgery, I never *felt* like trying anything, so of course I didn't do well in anything. But this time it didn't bother me because I was trying. . . .

"The chance to try has been very important to me. I've seen so many people who say "I can't" when they haven't even tried. Maybe their reasons are good, but if it's the fear of defeat, that isn't good. You can't open yourself to the chance for a victory without the possibility of defeat.

"At the end of my freshman year, I tried out for cheerleading and. . .made it!. There I was, probably the shyest person at school, and for two years I jumped around in front of a crowd like I honestly belonged there. . . .I must admit. . .there were a few times when a lot of tape eased a few worries.

"I've been in gymnastics now for four years. . . . I'd seen Cathy Rigby whipping around those bars and I wasn't so sure how well my stoma was going to like that. I told my coach I had an ileostomy and I didn't know if there would be any trouble or not. She said, simply, 'That's okay, just don't do anything that gives you trouble.'

". . . Well, I'm no great gynmast, there are a lot of things I can't do, but there's nothing I can't do because of my stoma. . .

"Besides a strong love for the excitement of being a gymnast, it's those strangers whom I came to know and love after my surgery, the ones who said, 'You can, Lori, You can!' And the fact that I can *try*. I fall and come home with new bruises all the time, but I can try!

"As far as my stoma is concerned, well, without it, I wouldn't have those voices implanted in my mind that drive me to higher goals. And more important than that, I wouldn't be alive to try."

Sports offer something for everyone: for the person who prefers gentle exercise in private and for those who like the companionship of shared sports, competitive or noncompetitive. There's a sport for everyone—from miniature golf to skin diving.

Barbara Hurewitz of the Ileostomy Association of New York had always wanted to try fencing, but her chance didn't come until after her ileostomy: "I was worried at first about the idea of a sword piercing my appliance, but this proved to be an imaginary fear. If you wear a long fencing jacket or even a sweater, you are more than adequately protected against a fencing foil."

Barbara also recommends dancing as a sport but warns beginning dancers to go easy on abdominal stretches and exercises at first. For dancers, she suggests a dance tunic or a short dance skirt over a leotard for women, a short tunic over briefs for men.

Belly dancing used to be called 'the only activity closed to ostomates,' but Jo Madsen of Eureka, California — who also happens to be a grandmother — belly dances for special events. She also practices yoga, runs two miles a day, and swims as often as she can. As a frequent traveler, she often startles stewardesses when she continues her habit of daily headstands even on the airplane, sometimes in the aisle!

Ellen P. Fincher of Orange County, a born athlete, joyously started horseback riding at 13 but was soon stopped by a long two-year fight with ulcerative colitis. However, within a year after her surgery she was riding again, and also found time to get married and find a job. Now she and her husband participate in equestrian events three weekends a month, saving the fourth for meetings of the Orange County Ostomy Association!

Most ostomates have no special problems skiing. One who does — but has found ways to overcome them — is Larry Kunz of Colorado. Born with a severe spinal defect, Larry can barely walk and has minimal control of his legs and feet. He had a urinary diversion when he was six years old. After moving to Colorado from New York, he took up skiing. His instructor, Hal O'Leary, had established a special ski program for people with physical disabilities, but had never taught anyone with *spina bifida*. Excited at first, Larry became discouraged:

"It was really, really tough. But then one day, Hal started yelling at me, 'Do you want to be a cripple all your life?'

That was the turning point."

Now Larry can sky any slope, any sort of terrain. He uses "outriggers," crutch-like devices with ski bottoms, instead of conventional poles, and he schusses the slopes with the tips of his skis tied together by a six-inch length of nylon.

"That's to keep me from doing the splits and hurting myself," explains Larry. "And if I'm going to race, I tie them even closer together."

For all ostomates contemplating a return to or a first try at a sport, there are a few common sense reminders:

Check with your doctor first. He can advise you on any limitations imposed either by your surgery or your general condition.

Pick a sport that sounds like fun to you. If all your friends are jogging but you loathe the idea, try something else. Bernice Kaufman Ordover advises that "Exercise should be relaxing, comfortable and fun! . . . Most people put themselves into a rigid exercise program, get sore muscles and give it up. They punish themselves and then their body rejects it. Try dancing at home to your favorite music. Jog when you walk the dog. Use your legs and not the wheels of your car."

Take it easy at first. Getting utterly exhausted during your first session will only make you discouraged and unnecessarily sore. Building muscles and endurance slowly works better for any prospective athlete, ostomate or not.

Use the right equiment. This goes not only for equipment specific for each sport — like comfortable jogging shoes for joggers or proper protective equipment for football players—but for ostomy equipment as well. Security during active movement is your goal. A little trial and error plus some advice from other sport-minded ostomates help. You may want to switch from your regular equipment, perhaps add a belt, try a panty girdle or close-fitting jockey shorts. All that activity, heat, and perspiration may make more frequent appliance changes necessary. And it makes sense to start out with an empty appliance. Don't forget to replace all those fluids lost in perspiration. After all, Gatorade® was developed for athletes.

Plysical Education major Karen Koehler, from New York, includes softball, basketball, volleyball, hockey, golf, archery, badminton and tennis in her college regimen. Her ostomy did cause her a problem once. In the third quarter of an "away" basketball game (with her team a few points behind) vigorous play plus a collision with an opponent caused her appliance to loosen. Quickly she asked the referee to excuse her from the game for medical reasons, dashed to the locker room, and used her emergency kit. She was back in the game in time for the fourth quarter—and in time to score the winning three points!

Keep playing. It takes time for all the benefits of a sport to show. Regular exercise pays far more dividends in terms of health, looks, and energy than intense sporadic spurts, alternating with bouts of inertia.

Most of all, *enjoy it.*

What gymnast Lori Musser says is worth repeating: ". . . There are a lot of things I can't do, but there's nothing I can't do because of my stoma. . . ."

CHAPTER 23 ❋ *The Other Side of the World*

After surgery, they think they're never going to be able to travel again, not even from San Francisco to Colma, just twenty miles away! Then pretty soon —maybe six months later —I get a beautiful picture postcard from this patient, saying "Wish you were here," and it's postmarked Tokyo or someplace else—they're off on a 45-day cruise!

(From a conversation with Jean Alvers, ET, San Francisco)

Far from stopping people from traveling, ostomies seem to act as mysterious catalysts that send them on their way! Ostomates go *everywhere* — from backpacking in the Sierra to grand tours of Europe, traveling by foot, bicycle, horseback, car, boat, plane, roller skates, and camel back.

Many of us take that scary first trip after surgery just to prove it can be done. Then, bitten by the travel bug, some of us keep on going. This *is* an exciting world, and ostomates, whether freed from misery for the first time in years, or given a new chance at life —and some new priorities for living—want to see it all.

Perhaps not *everyone* is as adventurous as Esther E. Komarend of Boston. "It was March, 1970—the decision for an ileostomy was made. All my dreams of traveling to far-away places went out my mind. . . .[but] as the months rolled by and good health returned, I was ready for a 10-day trial visit to Copenhagen and to Stockholm in October, 1971—for I had a wonderful holiday and no problems. . . .February, 1971—I left on a 47-day trip, touring Africa from Dakar to Capetown, an exciting Safari, and then on to Addis Ababa. It was a perfect vacation! I enjoyed good health, 26,000 miles of safe flying, no ileostomy problems; however, I carried home five extra pounds. . . .February, 1973 — I went 'Around the World in 68 Days.' I visited 17 countries, flew 19,600 air miles on 29 airplanes, rode on an elephant and camel, glided in a canoe over rapids, found myself on dugouts, sampans, junks, walked about 140 miles, climbed hundreds of stairs, and enjoyed all the excitement that went with all of it. . . .After suffering from ulcerative colitis for twelve years, the ileostomy surgery I so dreaded has really made my life more beautiful. . . .Where next?"

Burt and Thelma Blanchard of Glendale, California, use ten-speed bikes instead of airplanes or elephants (although they fly or take the train to their take-off point). In 1976, on bikes, they followed the 1804-1806 Lewis and Clark Trail for some 600 miles from Missoula, Montana, to Portland, Oregon.

After Burt's ileostomy surgery in 1964, *and* recovery from a major heart attack in 1972, the Blanchards knew they needed regular exercise and, with the doctor's approval, chose biking. Beginning with short rides around the neighborhood, they started reaching out with more miles and overnight trips. In 1975, this over-fifty couple enjoyed a two-week biking vacation, exploring the San Juan Islands of Puget Sound. That convinced them that "as long as we were well prepared, we could handle just about any kind of bike tour." Inspired by success, they began training for that Lewis and Clark Trail ride.

It makes sense to wait until you've bounced back from surgery, and are reasonably comfortable with your stoma, before setting out. To gain confidence, many ostomates suggest short trips first. For instance, George A. McConney of Kalamazoo, Michigan, reports:

"When my urostomy was six months old, I took it to Chicago for an overnight stay. How simple that sounds, but how far from simple it was to me at that time! . . .The thought of going far away from my own bathroom, and sleeping in a strange bed was frightening. I packed enough equipment to last me for two weeks and we set out.

"With beginner's luck, nothing happened!" After completing his business, there was time for sight seeing, and for reflection: "Probably nothing before or since has done more to reconcile me to my urostomy than this trip without any problems."

After a similar dry run, the world's your oyster. . . .

Inspired by the overnight trip to Chicago, the McConneys decided they not only could travel but must:

"Surviving these difficulties, we tramped the streets of Rome, Florence, Venice and Naples and had a wonderful time. It was kind of a honeymoon. . . .I came home feeling that I could do anything I had done before my operation.

"The period that followed our return home was a tremendous letdown. Bags came unstuck day and night. This produced a general demoralizaion. It was also a period of particular stress at work. I began to feel that I could only function properly when on vacation!"

Acting on this intuition, the McConneys have since gone across the U.S. to Mexico, the West Coast and British Columbia, Central America, Greece and Turkey.

Other ostomates and ETs delight in sharing travel tips, along with their photographs and suntans. Here are some favorites:

First, *have a wonderful time*! You may face a few new challenges (as most travelers do), but, if you pack your sense of humor along with other necessities, they won't stop you.

Think ahead. Before you go, picture (as well as you can) the places you'll be and plan for privacy and security. For instance, one ostomate we know and her husband planned a cross-country drive to visit relatives who had a large house, a large family *and* just one bathroom. She decided to forget irrigating until she got home.

Instead, she took along a good supply of lightweight disposables so she wouldn't have to worry about any time limits on privacy.

Get any prescriptions needed — or recommendations for non-prescription drugs. Many ostomates, like many normally-plumbed people, will want a remedy for diarrhea; colostomates may wish to pack a mild laxative. If you're heading for a hot humid climate, you may want prescriptions for a fungicide to deal with any fungus problems around the stoma; the doctor or ET can give you instructions for using it. Foresighted ileostomate travelers to areas where tourist diarrhea is common pack some potassium chloride powder for electrolyte replacement drinks.

For any extensive trip, have prescriptions filled before you go. Some states and foreign countries do not honor prescriptions from your home state. Make a note of the generic name of each medicine (the drug's name without a registered trademark; *triamcinolone acetonide*, for instance, is the generic name for Kenalog®) in case of emergencies, and take along your doctor's name, address and phone number.

A "do not disturb" sign is helpful. Many colostomates swear by a package of clip-on metal shower curtain hooks. These can be made into a chain of any length for hanging irrigation equipment from shower curtain rod, shower head or any sturdy (not a suction) hook.

If you're traveling in the U.S. or Canada, bring along the latest list of all UOA chapters (published as a pull-out section each year in the Winter issue of *Ostomy Quarterly*) in case you need help finding a pharmacy, physician, ET or just another ostomate to talk to. The American on Canadian Cancer Society may also have information. If you're going abroad, check with the International Ostomy Association (c/o UOA) to locate groups in the countries you are visiting.

To sleep without worrying about accidents, pack a mattress cover of some type (it can be as simple as a large heavy plastic garbage bag to slip under the sheet). Water and cleansing agents in squeeze bottles make for pleasant, easy clean-ups along the way. Some travelers suggest packing your equipment at the time you are changing your appliance or irrigating, so you won't forget anything you need, whether your destination is Poughkeepsie or Rio de Janeiro.

Unless you're going only to places with a sure source of supply, take more supplies than you think you'll need. Be generous. Make a note of the name, size, order number and manufacturer of your basics and, just in case, take along the name and phone number of your appliance supplier. Many emergencies could be avoided by a quick call home and the speedy service of United Parcel.

Keep your supplies with you, or at least enough for 48 hours. A flight or carry-on bag or a briefcase can hold toilet necessities and a change of underwear as well as ostomy supplies. Never check your supplies through. Be sure they don't go astray by keeping them within arm's reach.

Comfortable wash-and-wear clothes are a boon for any traveler, including the ostomate. And while an extra change of clothing may make your suitcase a trifle heavier, it can increase your confidence.

A Medic-Alert emblem or an emergency card belongs with you at all times, but especially when you travel. You can use a commercially available warning or make your own with the vital information on it: what kind of an ostomy you have, any kind of medicine you are taking, and any special precautions (no enemas or rectal temperatures, for instance). Include a warning: "Do not remove surgical appliance without doctor's orders."

Take it easy with what you eat and drink. Although digestive upsets are most often associated with foreign countries, they can follow a Chinese meal in San Francisco, a bowl of chili in Texas, or a double slab of pecan pie a la mode in Atlanta, particularly for a recent ostomate whose system is still used to simpler or smoother fare.

Some ostomates find they can eat anything and everything, and that's one of the pleasures of travel. Julia Schreier of Flushing,

New York, has some wonderful gastronomic memories: "During the four strenuous weeks of go-go-going, not one bellyache, not one bout of indigestion or diarrhea did I experience. Indeed, I ate much more adventurously than my non-handicapped husband, drawing the line only at heavily spiced foods. Through two more subsequent trips, I have enjoyed broiled trout with platters of French fries in Geneva, spaghetti and meat sauce in Florence, cassata and gelati in Rome, Wiener schnitzel and pastry in Vienna, smoked salmon in Copenhagen, fish and chips in London, broiled scampi in a restaurant overlooking Michaelangelo Square, cantaloupe and salade in Paris, and wine with my dinner everywhere."

In case of tourist diarrhea (a problem for many travelers who've never heard of an ostomy), take your anti-diarrhea medication and stick to low-residue foods such as rice, soda crackers and bananas. Most important, drink *large* amounts of fluid to make up for the water and electrolyte loss: bouillon, tea with sugar, ginger ale. One basic drink calls for one quart of water mixed with one teaspoon salt, ½ teaspoon baking soda, ⅜ teaspoon potassium chloride powder and four teaspoons sugar or white Karo® syrup. Remember, an increase in fluids does not increase ostomy output for colostomates and ileostomates. Only urine output increases; the kidneys take care of balancing the body fluids.

Remember, too, those wise words of Satch Paige: "If your stomach disputes you, lie down and pacify it with cool thoughts."

For ileostomates and colostomates with loose stools, dehydration occurs frequently and insidiously, especially during long car rides or summer traveling. Watch for weakness, thirst, decreasing urination. Better yet, prevent dehydration by drinking plenty of water and/or electrolyte-rich drinks. An immersion rod, a mug and a jug of water make fine hot drinks with tea bags, coffee and cocoa.

Expect the unexpected. That usually well-mannered colostomy or reasonably docile ileostomy may act up a bit. The colostomy may require a drainable appliance for a day or two instead of a gauze square. Relax. Such troubles are usually temporary and, meanwhile, you're on your way!

For *campers*, *motorists*, *airline and international* travelers, there are some more specific hints:

Campers rough it in varying degrees. Those who have self-contained recreational vehicles need make few adjustments for ostomies. Experienced campground campers suggest bringing plenty of toilet paper as well as aluminum foil (or opaque plastic bags) for disposing of used appliances. A waterproof rectangular plastic storage box (perhaps the kind meant to crisp celery and carrots in your refrigerator) works well both for storing supplies and for soaking reusable appliances. To avoid a chilly 3 a.m. trip to an outdoor privy, a number of campers suggest lining a large coffee can with a plastic bag, covering it with its own plastic lid and keeping it in your tent.

Victoria Campigotto from Ohio reports meeting another irrigating colostomate in a camp bathhouse about five o'clock in the morning:

"...There was a woman at the basin filling a colostomy irrigation bag and a one-half gallon thermos jug with warm water." After Victoria admitted to her new friend that 'I never had the nerve or the know-how to do it this way,' the woman showed her the equipment she had brought in her basket-type purse: regular paraphernalia plus water jug, a plastic funnel and a bent coat hanger which she bent into an over-the-door hook, with the hanger hook down, on which she hung her irrigating bag.

Ranging farther into the wilderness, ostomates continue to cope, using portable toilets with perhaps a tarp hitched between trees for privacy. Extremes in temperature cause some problems for karaya and other seals, and may mean more frequent changes. A cooler works well for storage; a few drops of warm water will restore seals that are too cold. Major changes in altitude may puff up plastic bottles storing cleaning supplies; squeezing out all the air before packing helps.

Veteran traveler Elnore Sturm, ET, LVN, from St. Louis, tells of her experience on a 200-mile boat trip down the Colorado River with a group of 16 people. An ileostomate who switched to disposable equipment for the trip, she worried beforehand about maintaining her appliance. No bother! A portable chemical toilet placed behind a large boulder away from camp, together with a series of signals for when it was in use, provided relief for everyone, not just Elnore, during the night. But: "The day was another story. We were instructed to drink plenty of water to remain hydrated as the temperature can get as high as 115 degrees and also were told that this would lead to 'pit' stops but would be no problem. We would have to ask to pull to the side when possible (on a small sand bar with some bushes or large rocks for privacy) and were to ask for the shovel, paper and matches! . . . I had to ask for a few extra stops, but no one except my husband really knew why! Colostomates would not be able to irrigate but would have to let nature take its course like the rest of the gang."

For traveling by car, seatbelts are safest when worn above or below the stoma; a long trip with a seatbelt rubbing the stoma directly may lead to irritation. But do wear them. As one doctor says, "I'd much rather fix an irritated stoma than massive internal injuries."

Glove compartments and trunks are usually too hot for supplies; a cooler or any place out of the sun works better. Since not all highway rest rooms are well equipped, carry tissue, soap, hand towels, and wash cloths. An unscented spray deodorant or a few drops of appliance deodorant can show thoughtfulness in car or public restroom. Cloth appliance covers or even a large soft handerchief placed between appliance and skin makes for cooler, more comfortable traveling. So does talcum powder. And this is definitely the time to use that favorite cushion.

Air travel presents its own challenges. Ostomates who wear metal faceplates may want to bring an extra faceplate and/or a doctor's statement to show security guards at the metal detector. You can request a private custom's inspection if you wish.

Small quantities of inflammable cements and solvents for medical purposes can now be carried on a plane; many ostomates choose non-flammable kinds for air travel, however. Remember to empty ileostomy and urostomy appliances long enough before takeoff and landing to forestall ending up in a long line at the restroom. Emptying pouches relatively frequently while in flight also avoids problems, as does expelling air carefully from appliances and any tubes or plastic bottles of cement before takeoff.

Cross-country air travelers face the problem of jet lag, although not as severely as round-the-world travelers do. It's possible that a normally well-behaved colostomy may lag along with the rest of you. A day or so of adjustment to the new time zone should bring you back to a more normal schedule. Some people prefer to anticipate time zone changes, starting to change their irrigation schedule about a week beforehand if they irrigate. Some recent reports indicate that dehydration may contribute to jet lag. One jet plane crew suggests drinking a glass of water every hour you're in a jet plane to counteract dehydration caused by cabin pressurization.

International boundaries prove no bar to ostomates. Carol Norris, of Eureka, California, tells of a year in Australia with her botanist husband, Dan, who was on sabbatical. After her surgery for a brief but brutal bout with ulcerative colitis and peritonitis, "ghoulish friends 'prepared' me never to be able to teach, dance, swim, or travel again. To prove them wrong, I did all those things, and added tenting. We camped from British Columbia to Newfoundland to Mexico and I toured Europe, sleeping with a girlfriend in a VW squareback. The Australia-Fiji year meant tenting for most of 40,000 miles, except for a few months in flats or cabin en route. . . . I never sprang a leak, though I swam in the jellyfishy Coral Sea, slept on buses and slid down cliffs. Our wee tent became a snug home when things went 'bump,' 'screech,' 'thapthapthap' and 'heeheehahee' in the rainforests."

Between writing novels and guides for the deaf, Carol has added thousands more miles to her travel logs, including a summer from Scotland to Finland, quick visits to New York to see her agent and botanical expeditions in Death Valley.

Sandra Zarcades, of Del Mar, California, faced with the chance to live in Greece for a year, at first doubted her ability to cope: "My imagination conjured up a whole series of problems that could plague me: a terrible heat wave, intestinal flu, food blockage, and bouts of diarrhea." She reports a wonderfully stimulating year despite a few problems. She learned to sample new foods very cautiously. Because of hot climate, she always carried a canteen with her for shopping excursions and for walking tours, drinking from it frequently. An ileostomate, she discovered new sources of potassium for herself in a country where frozen orange juice and bananas are rare: tomatoes in the summer and broccoli in the fall supplemented other foods.

International travelers have many resources they can call on. The International Association for Medical Assistance to Travelers (IAMAT), 350 - 5th Avenue, New York, New York 10001, provides information on doctors, hospitals and such. For details and costs, phone or write, enclosing a stamped, self-addressed envelope. The American Embassy, a Consulate, or a U.S. Military hospital in each country is another possible resource.

Get any prescriptions you need filled before you go (including one for an anti-diarrheal), and carry them with you in the original labeled containers (to avoid confusing customs inspectors on the look-out for illegal drugs). Prescriptions should carry the generic name of the medicine or its formula, since other countries may have different brand names for a drug if you need a refill.

Get any necessary shots well before bon voyage time, so any reactions will be well behind you when you leave.

What about water for irrigation or cleaning, as well as for drinking? A good rule of thumb is that anything that can go into your mouth can go into your stoma; but even clean water may contain bacteria that are unfamiliar to our systems. When there is any doubt, boil water (unless you are at a high altitude). Or purify it by adding to 1 quart of water either (a) 1 or 2 tablets of Halizone,

(b) 2% tincture of iodine (5 drops if water is clear, 10 drops if water is cloudy), or (c) 10 drops of chlorine bleach—mix and let stand 30 minutes. In an emergency, travelers have used bottled mineral water or even beer for irrigating and report they work fine. (Leave any carbonated drink out overnight to remove the carbonation bubbles.)

One point for international travelers over 65: Social Security Medicare does not cover health care expenses outside the U.S. It might be well to take out private health insurance for the duration of the journey. Contact your medical insurance company or the Passport Office for further information.

On the lighter side, *The Town Karaya*, a Nevada ostomy newsletter, suggests using an extra ostomy pouch on self or mate, as a money belt!

So, whatever your destination, plan ahead, use the resources available to you, meet each moment as it comes, and bring back a few hints of your own to share with other ostomates.

And—have a wonderful time!

CHAPTER 24 �֍ *Enterostomal*
Therapy: A New Profession

When a surgeon rearranged her personal plumbing some 25 years
ago, Norma Gill had no intention of getting into the profession of
enterostomal therapy. For one thing, there was no such
profession. . . .

Norma Gill was one of the ostomy pioneers. As a young
housewife in Akron, Ohio, pregnant with her third child, she
learned that she would need an ileostomy for her severe ulcerative
colitis. She already had some unhappy notions about ostomies
since her grandmother (at 74) had had a colostomy for cancer a few
years before. It had been impossible to find ostomy equipment,
and Norma remembered her aunts dealing with clumsy piles of
dressings that never quite hid the odor.

At the time of her own surgery in 1954, Norma was bedridden
for many miserable months. "It was then that I made a vow to God
that if I ever got out of that mess I'd devote the rest of my life to
rehabilitation of ostomates." And that's exactly what Norma
Gill has done. First she made a name for herself as an ostomy
volunteer in Akron. Then her surgeon, Dr. Rupert Turnbull of
the Cleveland Clinic, learned of her interest. In 1958, he put her
to work helping his patients at the Clinic, and gave her new

specialty a name — enterostomal therapy (*entero:* intestine — *stoma:* opening). The term stuck; it's commonly abbreviated as ET. In spite of a thousand problems, the results were so successful that in 1961 Dr. Turnbull suggested they start a School of Enterostomal Therapy so other ostomates could learn how to help.

About the same time Norma Gill was learning her unexpected profession in Cleveland and starting to teach, other new ostomates around the country were not only telling themselves that "something must be done," but finding ways of doing it. Even before the Cleveland school officially opened, Bertha Okun arrived from Montreal determined to learn to be an ET. In San Francisco, Jean Alvers was a young housewife with some experience in business administration until her acute illness led to an ostomy. Although her surgeons did a fine job, they didn't know how to tell her to care for her new stoma, so Jean in desperation experimented with plastic bags from a delicatessen, some tape used on airplane wings and other oddments, until she'd invented an appliance that worked for her. Her doctors, amazed and impressed, started asking her to help other patients.

Meanwhile, in Boston, Edith Lenneberg took a different route after her ostomy. A music teacher with small children at home, she helped found the Boston Ostomy Association in 1952 and then, in 1957, became the editor of the first national journal for ostomates, *The Ileostomy Quarterly.* Along with news (including a profile of Norma Gill after her appointment as an enterostomal therapist), professional articles and tips, the *Quarterly* printed the names of new groups of ostomates as soon as they were formed, thus helping people find each other. That's how Jane Walker from Atlanta, Georgia, knew where to call after her ileostomy, when she wondered both how to manage and how she might help. Among other things, she became an ET, helped organize ostomy groups all over Georgia, and developed the first UOA liaison with the American Cancer Society.

Although they knew the mushrooming need, those ostomy

pioneers didn't have it easy in those early days. Thanks to such medical breakthroughs as antibiotics and better transfusion techniques, more and more patients were surviving ostomy surgery; it was no longer high-risk. However, advice on how to live with such changes was almost non-existent. Appliances were cumbersome, inefficient, and hard to find. Hospitals didn't always take kindly to these newly-minted experts whose main prerequisite for training was neither an MD nor an RN, but a stoma. Many doctors and nurses ignored them as mavericks. And most patients, however much they needed them, didn't know that enterostomal therapists existed.

When, in 1962, the scatter of mutual aid groups around the country voted to join together and found the United Ostomy Association, the *Ileostomy Quarterly* suspended publication and the first issue of *Ostomy Quarterly* appeared in December, 1963. Edith finished the research project on ileostomy patients she'd started under a federal grant (from the then Office of Vocational Rehabilitation) while she was editor, saw the results published as a book, and then returned to music teaching until she was persuaded to open the Stoma Rehabilitation Clinic at New England Deaconess Hospital in Boston in 1967.

In 1968, Norma Gill and the growing number of ETs who attended the UOA conference in Phoenix, Arizona, were persuaded by Dr. Turnbull that they needed a firmer and more formal way to keep in touch than chance meetings, long-distance phone calls, and postcards. They formed the North American Association of Enterostomal Therapists, later renamed the International Association For Enterostomal Therapy (IAET). This organization would hold them together, allowing them to share information, set standards of practice and certify other schools for ET training. With such a professional approach, they hoped the medical profession would come to recognize their value.

At the banquet at the 1979 annual IAET Conference in Vancouver, B.C., the delegates toasted Norma Gill and put on a special program in honor of a teacher whose spunk and determination have had much to do with improving matters for ostomates everywhere. By the time of that banquet, there were over a thousand ETs in North America, no longer mavericks but welcome members of the health care team. Among them were Sally Gill Thompson, ET (Norma Gill's daughter) and Debbie Okun Shaikin, ET (Bertha Okun's daughter).

As ostomates discover, one by one, ETs fill an enormous gap. Most nurses are lucky if they have a two-hour lecture on ostomies during their training, and many have never seen a stoma. As for doctors, Mike Schreiber said: ". . . If [the surgeon] took the time to instruct each of his ostomy patients about ostomy care in minute detail, I wonder how many surgeries he would have to forego and how many lives might be sacrificed because he didn't have sufficient time to do the important surgical tasks he had been trained to do."

ETs know that — important as attitudes are — proper information about stoma care can mean the difference between a dreary, bitter life as a self-styled handicapped recluse, and a good full life as a normal person, eager to enjoy the new life an ostomy has made possible. The person with an ostomy needs to know about skin care and skin problems, the best appliances for a given stoma, techniques for irrigating if a colostomate chooses that option, and a host of other nitty-gritty matters. These technical aspects of ostomy care—as well as psychological aspects of coping —are the heart of the ET's domain.

Before surgery, ETs find time to explain what's going to happen, and why, and to reassure patients and their families that this surgery they may have never heard of before is not the end, but a new beginning. Alone or with the surgeon, they find and mark the best stoma site before surgery. After, they help the patient determine the best ways to cope with the new stoma, choose equipment, and learn how to manage and return to former activities and jobs. Along with this technical and practical know-how, there's empathy for the person adjusting to such changes, and a willingness to be called about minor (and major) problems.

Besides teaching and counseling patients, ETs also can and do teach doctors and nurses, giving in-service training programs and organizing regional workshops. In addition, some ETs are active in research, and many work closely with local UOA chapters.

As Bobbie Brewer (herself an ET) said, "The ET is more than a pouch changer. Much more. She (or he) is a rehabilitation worker in the fullest sense of that word, helping the patient return to a full life."

In spite of a thousand-fold increase in their ranks since 1958, geography still makes the services of an ET a luxury in many parts of the country. At Coos Bay on the Oregon Coast, for instance, the nearest ET is hundreds of miles away, so the local group arranged for an all-too-brief visit from a California expert. Even in urban areas, many hospitals still don't have an ET on the staff, and some still deny the necessity.

Since being a registered nurse is now a prerequisite for ET training—and a stoma is not—many ETs do not have ostomies themselves. Some have been attracted to the field because of the experience of a close family member or a friend. Others are recruited by hospitals from the ranks of staff or are encouraged by the American and Canadian Cancer Societies or the local UOA group. Empathy for the person acquiring an ostomy is still an admission requirement for the ET candidate, with or without a stoma. (Non-ostomate ETs wear pouches full of water to see how that feels.)

Personal experience with ostomy surgery is still responsible for many recruits, including Melba Connors. She was already an RN when she opened her eyes after emergency surgery resulting from ulcerative colitis to find herself with an ostomy. She told about her experience in the *American Journal of Nursing:* "Depression settled like a fog, separating me from the figures who came in and out of the room."

People told her it would be easy because she was herself a nurse.

"'I'm not a nurse,' I screamed within myself. 'I'm a human being who is scared to death. I'm afraid my husband won't love me, my teenage children will reject me, and I'll smell bad and offend my friends. Help me!'"

Although her internist assured her that she could have a normal life, she did not believe him: "'Your idea of a normal life is different than mine,' I thought. 'I'll never wear tight clothes again. I'll have a restricted diet. How will I manage the care? Everyone who comes in takes care of it differently. . .!'"

As the hospital days dragged on and Melba encountered discomforts and complications — severe pain in the perineal wound, noise, non-stop gas, excoriated skin, a leaking appliance, and a roommate who called her "Stinky"—she plummeted deeper into depression, crying at night when she thought no one would hear.

Then, "One day the student nurse who was caring for me said casually, 'You know, my roommate has an ileostomy. Would you like to talk to her?' A student nurse with an ileostomy! 'Yes, of course, I'd like to see her.'

"Just after visiting hours, a darling young girl in a very tight, form-fitting dress walked in. 'Hi,' she said. 'I'm Sandy. My roommate said you would like to talk to me.' I was astounded. This vivacious, slim girl could not have an ileostomy! 'Sorry I'm late. I was just starved, so I stopped to pick up a pizza before I came.' A pizza! I thought of the horrible, bland diet I was eating and suspected she did not have a stoma at all."

She did, though, and her help in selecting an appliance as well as in showing what an ileostomate could do proved the turning point for Melba: "With this appliance, I no longer had sore skin or accidents, and the odor was controlled. By now I could see quite a bit of blue sky."

An article in a nursing journal led Melba to her specialty, for she remembers those first frustrations — and what a blessing a little help was. After working as an ET with the Visiting Nurse Program in San Diego, she became director of the Enterostomal

Training Program at the University of California, San Diego, School of Medicine.

Bonnie Bolinger, RN, ET, was drawn to ET training by her remembered anguish as a mother. When her daughter, Michelle, was six, she had to have a vesicostomy (a hard-to-manage type of urinary diversion). "The statement that registered most in my mind was, 'She will be the first child with the surgery in Dayton, Ohio.' Reassurance out the window—isolation to take its place.

"Isolation and lack of knowledge by the health care team left me wondering. Where was I to go for help? Who would understand my six-year-old's needs? Her goal was to enter first grade. The school didn't want her. The surgeon ordered equipment that would not fit an adult, much less a child.

"Anger, anger, anger at all concerned. Her vesicostomy looked crude, her abdomen appeared to have second degree burns, she hurt, I hurt, her father retreated, her brothers didn't understand all the tension and tears. I called my sister, an RN, and pleaded for her to take my first-born and relieve me of my anguish. My sister proceeded to wrap Michelle in a blanket and storm every doctor's office that had been involved with the case, demanding action.

"She got action! Three doctors called within two hours. Equipment was ordered and Mr. Botvin from Torbot Company taught me to care for Michelle over the phone. He conveyed knowledge, reassurance, and a hot-line number for follow-up care."

ET training came later when Michelle was 12 and the other children had reached school age. Though Bonnie wasn't sure she could handle the courses, she went first to school to become a licensed vocational nurse. ET school came later, as did becoming an RN. Bonnie, like her daughter, was also a first—the first ET in Dayton, Ohio. She's delighted with the way attitudes toward ostomies have changed in recent years and became President of IAET.

Gerry Cameron, RN, ET, doesn't have a stoma. However, when

she began the Patient Education Department at Queen of the Valley Hospital in Napa, California, she was concerned about the lack of information for people who'd had ostomies. At a regional UOA meeting in Sacramento, she heard for the first time about the nursing specialty of enterostomal therapy.

For three months she pondered how she could manage the training, and then talked it over with her husband. He said she should apply in spite of many obstacles. These seemed to disappear like magic. Her best friend's folks lived in San Diego; she could stay with them. The American Cancer Society provided the money. Her husband's cousin came to look after the family for the six weeks she'd be away, and her husband drove with her to San Diego, flying home and leaving her the car.

Gerry found the training very interesting. Since completing it, ". . . it has been my pleasure to work with many people with ostomies. Each one is a special person to me, and I continue to find my work a very rewarding experience."

Eunice Gaskell, RN, ET, was head nurse on a surgical floor of a Modesto hospital. "I realized ostomy patients seemed frustrated, even with the teaching after surgery, so I told them to call me after they were home and had a problem. The phone calls began. So did the idea of further education and selling a program to the hospital and physicians. One of the satisfactions, since I've had my ET training, is being able to work with the patients and their families in the hospital and after discharge for continuity of care."

More than a dozen approved schools now offer programs leading to certification as enterostomal therapists. In spite of high admission requirements, waiting lists are long. Requirements vary from school to school but, in general, applicants must be RNs with at least two years clinical experience in the last five years. They also need high recommendations and must have a job waiting for them with a sponsoring hospital or organization in their home communities. The programs offer six to eight weeks of intensive training, clinical and academic. In a few cases, training programs have been incorporated into Master's Degree programs in nursing. For a list of schools, write to International Association for Enterostomal Therapy, 505 N. Tustin St., Suite 219, Santa Ana, CA 92705.

What do ET students learn? Working with many specialists— colon and rectal surgeons, dermatologists, dietitians, gastroenterologists, oncologists, social workers, discharge co-ordinators, psychiatrists, and ETs, to name a few — students learn the anatomy and physiology of the many different kinds of ostomies. They observe surgery, learn to care for patients from before surgery through the hospital experience, discharge and beyond, teach patients, other health professionals and the general public, and attend meetings of local UOA chapters. Lectures alternate with observation and clinical practice. Supervision is close. It is almost an apprenticeship program, since most schools limit enrollment to a few students at a time.

In the early days, ETs not only wondered whether they dared charge for their services but financed their training themselves. Now, hospitals sometimes pay for training of a selected staff member. Both the American Cancer Society and Canadian Cancer Society often help. So do local UOA chapters. In addition, IAET offers a scholarship, funded by commercial ostomy suppliers, and the United Ostomy Association has established the Archie Vinitsky Scholarship for Enterostomal Therapy.

As for fees, Bobbie Brewer explains, "The ET expects to be treated by the patient as a professional, not as a social contact, and to be called for an appointment and to bill for services rendered." Some insurance plans cover ET services; some do not.

After passing the certification exam, the new ET returns home to a waiting job — working in a hospital, for several hospitals, with home care groups like Visiting Nurse Association, or in a stoma rehabilitation clinic. Private practice is another option, and some ETs are employed by appliance manufacturers. A new book by Linda Gross, ET, and Zeila Bailey, RN—*Enterostomal Therapy: Developing Institutional and Community Programs* (Nursing Resources, Inc., 1979) explores some of the options. After joining

IAET, the ET has further resources, including refresher courses, annual conferences and the professional journal, *The Journal of Enterostomal Therapy.*

Although the outlook for the rehabilitation of ostomates in the United States and Canada has improved dramatically in a handful of years, other countries are not as fortunate. The number of trained stomal therapists is increasing in England and Australia, but the rest of the world still has only a handful, along with some special problems. In a developing country, for instance, where a multi-generational family of eight or more may share one room, privacy is impossible. Sanitary facilities and appliances may be non-existent. Attitudes and cultural norms can also create problems. Prilli Stevens, RN, ET from Capetown, South Africa, reports that she's called "Bad Lady" by witch doctors who harass her.

In many countries, importing ostomy appliances and supplies is a problem because of prohibitive duties, bureaucratic hassles, and high taxes. (In India, for example, only a doctor can import ostomy supplies.) Together with the International Ostomy Association, the World Council of Enterosomal Therapists is fighting such problems.

UOA and IAET are growing up together. Trained UOA visitors and ETs complement each other and, once in a while, conflict. A decade or two ago, visitors from the local ostomy group—if one existed—were the only resource to help patients, so visitors gave the best answers they could to questions about appliance choice, skin care, and other matters. Margot Julian, RN, ET (and an ileostomate from the San Francisco Bay Area who has been active in UOA at both local and national levels) explains how roles have changed:

"An ET is a trained specialist, usually a nurse, whose profession is planning the rehabilitation of those who have had surgical diversion of the bowel or bladder. This involves counseling on the psychosocial aspects as well as the selection of prosthetic devices and instructions on their use. . . .

"The certified visitor is an ostomate who has been carefully selected and trained to 'help establish the patient's graceful acceptance of the stoma and speed his return to normal living.' Visitors should not give medical advice, provide nursing care, nor attempt to practice enterostomal therapy. Visitors can give something that can never be provided by a non-ostomate: living proof that there *is* life after surgery. . . .

"Through the years, in recognition of the fact that behind every stoma is a whole patient with other nursing needs, and for legal reasons, enterostomal therapy has evolved into a nursing specialty. The emergence of the enterostomal therapist released the ostomy visitor from the responsibility of providing advice on stoma management. This is an increasingly complex task as the technology improves its response to needs of ostomates largely as expressed through the UOA. At the same time, the trend toward non-ostomate RN-ETs makes it imperative that good visitors be available to do what they do best, to provide moral support on a one-to-one basis from someone who has 'been there.'"

The hours are long and the work is hard, but most ETs find great satisfaction in their jobs.

All too often, in addition to helping the new ostomate, they must still rescue long-time ostomates who've had no advice on how to manage or instructions so hurried the patient didn't understand. Melba Connors comments on some of the repair work an ET runs into:

"I have visited people who had bought appliances over the counter in a surgical supply house. Leaking and odor were borne with stiff upper lips. They have never complained about their horrendous skin irritations . . . because they thought that everyone that had this surgery had the same problems."

Melba also tells a harrowing story about a woman who'd had a colostomy for twenty years. After surgery, she was taught to irrigate with a standard enema set-up and for 20 years had been confined to her home, using 10 quarts of water and spending six hours a day in the bathroom, lying over the toilet. "Fortunately, in one lesson, I was able to modify her equipment so that a dam could be used, provide her with an irrigating sleeve and the correct method of irrigation, using one quart of water. . . . By the end of the week she had control and she was able to throw away her pouch forever. With tears in her eyes she thanked me for rescuing her from bondage. The tears in my eyes, though, were for the never-to-be-recovered 20 years that she had lost."

CHAPTER 25 ✻ *The Phoenix:* *UOA and Its Ancestors*

How beauteous mankind is! O brave new world, That has such
people in 't!
Shakespeare, *The Tempest*

No bells rang, no trumpets blared that February in 1949 when a handful of ostomates met in a hospital room near Philadelphia. They had no inkling that this would be the beginning of a movement which would sweep the United States, Canada and, eventually, the world.

They weren't concerned with triumphs of the future, but with solving immediate problems. "Successful" ostomy surgery had left them with intolerable problems: skin breakdown, primitive appliances, and odor, among others. Worse still was the sense of isolation, of being different from everyone else. The name of the hospital — Valley Forge — seemed singularly appropriate. Like General Washington and his troops almost two centuries before, the ostomates were facing a Valley Forge of illness, desolation, and near-despair.

Now they had found each other. Sharing experiences and problems, they found solutions sometimes, moral support always.

That was the beginning. The late Ira Karon, a past president of the United Ostomy Association, wrote about the next steps: "...In February of 1950 the second group was formed in Los Angeles, and in 1951 QT New York came into being. These groups were formed, each without knowledge of other and each was begun at the suggestion of a surgeon."

In the case of QT New York, the surgeon was Albert S. Lyons (who has worked closely with UOA ever since). Aware that his ileostomy patients were surviving surgery—but barely surviving the aftermath—he and hospital social worker Miss Lucy Neary set up a meeting of ileostomate women from Ward T of Mt. Sinai Hospital, New York City. At the third get-together, in the social work office at Mt. Sinai, 15 people showed up, including male ileostomates from Ward Q. Thus began QT New York. Dr. George Schreiber joined QT in its first months. (Both doctors faced the scoffs of other doctors who didn't like the idea of mutual-help groups for patients.) Within a few months, members were visiting new ileostomates in the hospital. A joint venture of QT New York and QT Boston, *QT Bulletin*, the first ostomy newsletter in the country, appeared early in 1952. That same year, Dr. Lyons and Dr. Schreiber opened the first stoma clinic in the nation, and Dr. Lyons wrote a letter, published in the *Journal of the American Medical Association*, about the success of this group approach.

New groups were springing up across the country: Boston, St. Paul, Minnesota, and elsewhere. In May, 1956, the first country-wide conference met in New York, with representatives from ten groups. Despite a push for unification, many representatives were reluctant to gather ileostomy and colostomy groups under a single banner. Participants relished their autonomy, but decided to keep in touch by publishing two national journals, one for colostomates and one for ileostomates. *The Ileostomy Quarterly*, edited by Edith Lenneberg of QT Boston, thrived (except financially); later it would become the *Ostomy Quarterly*. (The

Quarterly was exchanged in bulk across the Atlantic for copies of the publication of the Ileostomy Association of Great Britain, an organization formed in 1956; not only in America was the ostomy mutual-help movement gathering steam.)

The time was not yet ripe for unification in 1956. There were too many worries about whether ileostomates and colostomates could really help each other, too many fears about losing local independence and control.

But the dream of unification did not die. Sam Dubin, a small, quiet, and gentle man who had suffered from ulcerative colitis for years before his ileostomy in 1952, became standard bearer for the dream: a national organization to weld local ostomy groups into a powerful force for all ostomates. He infected others with his commitment to a united association for mutual aid, moral support, education and communication.

A second national meeting, late in 1960, brought together over 400 members in New York. Don Binder, who would later become Executive Director of UOA, drove all night from Cincinnati to attend: "We talked at the meeting about organizing a national association but nothing was resolved. When time ran out, some of us gathered that evening...to continue discussion....A steering committee was established, and they met the following year in Detroit to make further plans."

Archie Vinitsky, President of the St. Paul's Colostomy and Ileostomy Rehabilitation Guild, Inc., of Minnesota, led the Detroit meeting. Participants struggled to define purposes for a national organization—which local groups would accept. They decided that a national organization, without interfering with the aims and autonomy of the local chapters, "could act as a clearing-house of ideas and information for all clubs, could standardize a visiting program for greater helpfulness, could better reach the medical and lay public, could encourage research with greater financial resources, could stop wasteful duplication of effort, and could more effectively aid in the rehabilitation of people with ostomies." (Chairman Vinitsky would later serve as President of UOA; in the 1970s, he would guide the fledgling International Ostomy Association as its first President.)

Next stop was Cleveland, Ohio, for the Constitution Convention in 1962. Norma Gill, working full time at the Cleveland Clinic as the first stoma therapist, took on the task of organizing the Convention: "The first meeting in Cleveland was decided on at the last minute in Detroit when we all realized it was either now or never in forming a national association. Time doesn't permit [even mentioning] all our problems at that first convention, since there were no guidelines, no money and only our new Cleveland group."

Nevertheless, 115 representatives and six ostomy supply exhibitors attended the Convention on September 22, 1962. The name United Ostomy Association — Don Binder's suggestion — was accepted; national officers were elected. There was sadness too: in August, one month before his dream was to become a reality, Sam Dubin died of heart failure. In his memory, UOA would later name its highest honor the Sam Dubin Achievement Award.

The growing pains continued (and still do, as UOA keeps growing). Don Binder resumes the story: "My feeling when we left Cleveland was very doubtful that we would survive the first year. But 28 chapters affiliated and when we gathered the following September in Los Angeles for the 1st Annual Convention we had survived and had confidence that the Association would grow."

During this 1st UOA Annual Convention, the Board of Directors voted $2500 for publication of an international magazine devoted to ostomy problems. As Virginia Pearce Geiger (editor of the *Ostomy Quarterly* from its first issue, December 1963, until she resigned in 1978) recalls: "All jobs had to be done on a voluntary basis.

"Separated by over 2,000 miles and working in their spare time, the editor and business manager had to establish format, obtain copy and advertising, do the artwork, layout, printing and distribution of the magazine, plus solving a myriad of problems. However, without sufficient funds to finance the enterprise, the decision was made to proceed, because all concerned felt that the great need for such a publication far outweighed the obstacles to be overcome."

Those who were in at the beginning still catch their breath when they realize how far UOA has come. Dave Slutzky, for instance, one of the original group which met near Philadelphia in 1949, attended the 10th Annual Conference in San Francisco in 1972, where almost 1000 conferees gathered. He and the others listed as participants in the first national conference in 1956 — many of whom continue to serve, year after year, as the sturdy backbone of UOA — still find it hard to believe that the organization now numbers tens of thousands of members, in hundreds of chapters spanning the United States and Canada.

No matter how large it becomes, however, UOA cannot forget that it is a collection of local chapters. Each of these is a self-supporting unit with its own membership and officers. Monthly meetings, open to everyone, usually include a talk or panel discussion by doctors, nurses, and/or ostomates, along with displays of ostomy products, and plenty of discussion afterwards around the coffee pot, as experienced and novice ostomates get acquainted. Chapters publish their own newsletters, and encourage publicity in newspapers, radio, and television. With the help of medical advisors and enterostomal therapists, many chapters present in-service programs in hospitals.

Local chapters, often with the help of the local Cancer Society unit, train members to visit patients in hospitals and homes before and after ostomy surgery. Thousands upon thousands of ostomates remember that first breath of hope that blew in with a UOA visitor — smiling proof that a normal life was within reach after ostomy surgery. With the development of ETs well versed in technical know-how, UOA's Visitor Training Programs have changed. There's more concern about psychological support, less with "which bag is best."

As strength and health return, many new ostomates bring their questions and doubts to the local chapter meeting. And, as they become relative old-timers, many stay, passing on their experience and support to help newer ostomates.

The UOA is sectioned geographically into regions. A regional coordinator supervises other volunteers, who work directly with established chapters and develop new groups where they are needed. Each region holds an annual conference (called a conference rather than a convention to emphasize the educational programs and the seriousness of intent).

Regional programs dovetail snugly with the national program, which has headquarters in Los Angeles. National officers and a Board of Directors, all elected at the annual conference, decide on policy and new directions for UOA.

An executive director and a small staff oversee various administrative activities. UOA publishes booklets and guides on ostomy care (as well as the *Ostomy Quarterly*), and prepares charts, slides, and films. Among its activities, the national office guides national public relations, publicity, and fund-raising; keeps current membership lists and handles correspondence; coordinates the annual national conference which brings together ostomates, the medical professions and often spouses and children. While it does not have its own funds for research, UOA cooperates with organizations which do.

A professional advisory board includes doctors, ETs, pharmacists, and others to keep UOA abreast of new developments.

At the Constitution Convention in 1962, the delegates reluctantly (even apologetically, recalls Don Binder), asked for annual dues of 50¢. Although the fee has gone up a bit since then, it's still low. Local chapters collect dues, then send on a portion to the national office. Large gifts and grants are rare. Volunteer effort is what makes UOA survive—and thrive.

Why do people with ostomies even need such a group? Edith Lenneberg asked the question as part of a research project she conducted from 1958 to 1962: "Are they so immersed in self-pity that they need to withdraw and seek the company of commiserators; or does our society with its emphasis on 'normalcy' push them into a society-for-the-common-defense?" Edith concluded that ostomy and other mutual-help groups "...are the outgrowth of the increasing participation of the American public in matters of physical and emotional well-being...as a healthy effort at self-help towards the ultimate goal of...maximal self-dependence."

An ostomy group, thus, is a healthy step toward helping oneself—and then toward helping others. Together, ostomates have achieved what they could not have achieved alone. Without group pressure and ingenuity, most ostomates would still be grappling with a smelly, one-size-fits-all appliance, constantly reddened weepy skin, odor, and other problems. Worst of all, they would be *alone* in the struggle, without support and practical advice.

Thanks to the efforts of thousands of ostomates over many years, ostomy surgery, once considered "a fate worse than death," has become a chance for new life. To celebrate this rebirth "from the ashes of disease," UOA chose the phoenix as its symbol. Every five hundred years, this mythical, magical bird, knowing it is time to die, enters its nest of sweet-smelling myrrh, and rustles its glowing golden wings. The glow smolders into flame and the phoenix is consumed in a fiery holocaust. But as the glow fades, one spark rekindles, and then another — and from the ashes emerges the new phoenix: magnificent, towering, immortal.

Larry Litwack, the first president of UOA, wrote: "...The Phoenix represents a fiery symbol of the spirit and feeling underlying the growth of the Association. For the ostomate, what more appropriate choice could have been made? From the ashes of despair and disease, from the fear of disability and death, from the ebb tide of physical and emotional being to the full flood of life—of hope—of health. Reborn to a life of fulfillment—of dedication—of giving to others. Although not ourselves immortal as was the legendary bird, we gain perhaps true immortality by giving of ourselves to others, so that we live on forever in the hearts and minds of others."

Was it entirely a coincidence that the small town near Philadelphia where those first ostomates gathered in 1949—was Phoenixville?

CHAPTER 26 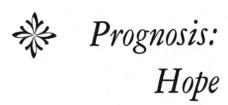 *Prognosis:*
Hope

*Edith Lenneberg is one ET who hopes her profession will begin to
self-destruct:*
*"Through earlier diagnosis, better medical treatment for
inflammatory bowel disease, research into diet and cancer, and
bringing the subject out in the open so people would not be afraid
to have little problems treated while they're still little, the
number of ostomies done each year could begin to drop. That
would be a lovely thing. In the meantime, I'm glad we are here
for those who need us."*

Many share Edith's dream. Around the world many are
working to make it come true.

A researcher in Baltimore spends long hours each day studying
the effects of different diets on the digestive tract. Do larger
amounts of fiber in the diet speed the passage of food through the
gut so that any cancer-causing substances don't get a foothold
there? How about the relative amounts of protein, carbohydrate
and fat in the diet — does that affect the intestine? Are there
specific foods or additives which seem to attack the digestive
tract? Are there any substances which protect the gut—perhaps
vitamins to keep the intestinal lining intact?

In San Francisco, another researcher looks at stress: what part, if any, does it play in the development of cancer or the inflammatory bowel diseases? Is acute stress the villain, or chronic stress—or do both play a role in disease? If stress is a factor, what can people do to protect themselves against its harmful effects?

In Atlanta, in Montreal, in London, other scientists struggle to unravel the riddles of the auto-immune diseases (which probably include Crohn's disease and ulcerative colitis), in which the body seems to attack part of itself. Is a virus at fault? What are the hereditary factors, if any? Are some personality types particularly vulnerable?

Still other researchers—those studying ways to prevent birth defects, for instance, or those wrestling with the causes of cancer — join the war on the diseases and problems which lead to ostomies.

Tackling the problem from another angle, doctors, nurses, health educators work to detect colo-rectal and bladder cancer at such an early stage that simple office procedures or minor surgery could eliminate it. They promote mass screening for hidden blood in the stool or urine, and sigmoidoscopies for adults over 50, tests which can find cancer in its infancy, can root it out before it has a chance to settle in. More sophisticated scopes for seeing the inside of the intestine and the bladder increase the chances for early diagnosis; polyps which may turn cancerous can be removed before they have a chance to cause trouble.

Those who publicize the need for such tests, in newspaper and magazine articles for example, make people aware of these tests. Publicity campaigns open the doors and windows on the matter of digestive and urinary tract problems. Then the fresh air of information and openness about this essential part of ourselves can blow away the cobwebs of fear and reticence.

Other health professionals participate in studies of alternate techniques for dealing with these diseases. Trials of different drugs for managing such problems as Crohn's disease last many years. Surgical ways to cope with urinary incontinence without an ostomy — the bladder pacemaker, for example — are future possibilities.

But until that happy day when the diseases and problems are wiped out or are all treated successfully without ostomy surgery, there will be plenty of ostomates around. Whatever the future brings, the number of ostomates *now* is large.

In the meantime, ostomy techniques and management change constantly. What seemed revolutionary a few years ago—like the continent ileostomy — is old hat now, and the prospects for continent ostomies for colostomates and urostomates get better every day. A few colostomates, for instance, have had a powerful magnetic ring implanted in the fatty layer around a flush stoma. This magnetic ring, wrapped in inert plastic, holds another metal magnetic disc firmly over the colostomy so that feces and gas cannot escape. When the person with such a device feels a sense of fullness, he goes to the bathroom, removes the outer cap, allows the feces to pass into the toilet, rinses or wipes with toilet tissue, and replaces the magnetic cap. If perfected, this magnetic ring and cap may mean more convenience for many colostomates.

Development of new materials, like the pyro-carbons (carbon powder processed under intense heat and pressure to make a substance which body tissues accept and even join) promises new possibilities of flap doors, valves and conduits that might replace appliances for some ostomates.

When there weren't many ostomates, there weren't many options either. But increasing numbers of ostomates led to greater demand for surgical improvements, better appliances, more individualized treatment. A vocal, organized, enthusiastic group of ostomates is, after all, pretty difficult to resist!

It hasn't taken long. From those beginnings in the 1950s, when isolated but energetic ostomates began to find each other and join forces, to today, is a very short time. But those few years have seen the formation and daily growth of the United Ostomy Association, the International Ostomy Association, the National

Foundation for Ileitis & Colitis, the International Association for Enterostomal Therapy, and the World Council of Enterostomal Therapists.

In 1975, the International Ostomy Association became the umbrella organization for ostomy groups all over the world. In England, in Nigeria, in India, around the globe, ostomates (or "ostomists" as they are called in England) are finding themselves no longer alone. IOA has some special priorities, besides helping individual ostomates and reaching the public with information about ostomies. Customs duties and import taxes, for example, remain hobgoblins, blocking the spread of appliances and products across some national borders.

Enthusiasm and good ideas from newer chapters around the world bubble over into longer-established chapters. Englishman Leslie F. Kingston, for instance, formed the Kingston Trust to set up homes where elderly "ileostomists" who could no longer look after their ostomies themselves would receive care. European chapters are encouraging their surgeons in pioneering techniques like the magnetic colostomy plug.

How much has changed! How short a time it has taken to go so far!

An ostomate in 1950, for instance, wore his one-size-fits-all appliance or a pile of pads, stayed at home most of the time, and wondered if he were the only one in the world to be in such a horrible condition. His stoma, poorly constructed by our current standards, would have proved unmanageable with the best of products. His skin was raw and oozing much of the time; constant leakage and odor kept him a recluse. There was no one to talk to, no one to share experiences with, no one to answer questions—and the aloneness and shame were perhaps the most painful parts of a miserable situation.

But the ostomate today faces a much sunnier prospect. Thanks to the ostomy visitor, the enterostomal therapist, friends (by telephone or letter, if necessary) in UOA, The *Ostomy Quarterly*, new surgical techniques, better appliances and skin care products, he can become not only healthy but "better than ever."

Karl Menninger, M.D. might have had ostomates in mind when he wrote: "Not infrequently we observe that a patient shows continued improvement past the point of his own 'normal' state of existence. He not only gets well, to use the vernacular; he gets as well as he was, and then he continues to improve still further. He increases his productivity, he expands his life and its horizons. He develops new talents, new powers, new effectiveness. He becomes, one might say, 'weller than well!'"

But there is much still to do.

The researcher in Houston working to conquer a condition which leads to an ostomy, the enterostomal therapist teaching a new ostomate in Bombay how to care for an appliance, the doctor in Chicago using a new type of colonoscope to snip out a polyp before it turns cancerous, a youth group in Santa Rosa sharing experiences, swapping stories—all are fighting on the same team.

With such tough and determined fighters, the prognosis *must* be hopeful.

CHAPTER 27 ❊ *In the Family*

When Mother phoned that March dusk in 1976, her spirits matched the weather outside.

Dismal.

She tucked in an alarming snippet of news near the end of a sprawling and woeful conversation: ". . . just a little bit of blood in my bowel movement. Probably nothing to worry about."

But she was scared. And so was I, despite my casual, "Yeah, probably not serious. Do keep an eye out though, just in case it happens again. Okay?"

Our fears crouched behind a veil of mutual reassurance. Never in my memory had Mother so much as mentioned the bowel — her's or anyone's.

And I? With two months to go before graduation from nursing school, I would have had to be a real dimwit not to have recognized the possible seriousness of such a complaint in a woman over 50 who'd never had even a whisper of trouble with her digestive tract.

A woman who happened to be very special to me.

Sure, it might be hemorrhoids. Maybe I was over-reacting. Maybe. . . .

A free-lance writer, Mother had little money and no doctor of her own. I confided my forebodings to a doctor friend who knew some of the community resources available. An appointment was arranged.

But Mother turned skittish. It took a few months and some cancelled appointments before she finally had the physical exam. I fumed and fussed. Patient's rights or no, sometimes I was tempted to hogtie her, if necessary, so long as she'd see the doctor.

We were both playing at make believe. To Mother, it was, as she would acknowledge later, a matter of "Until I see the doctor, there's nothing really wrong with me."

And I was striking my own bargain with Whomever had charge of these matters: if I just concentrated hard enough on the worst that could happen — the very worst — why then, it wouldn't happen. Simple as that.

In late June Mother finally had her physical. She was jubilant over the results, and so was the doctor.

Until that sigmoidoscopy a few days later. I had driven her to the appointment and sat outside the office. When I saw the doctor's face as he barreled out of his office and sprinted up the stairs (to get another doctor to take a look), I *knew*.

When the biopsy report came back a few days later, I had to *do* something, take some kind of action. I knew next to nothing about ostomies. I'd been "exposed" to the subject, by way of a brief and boring film two years earlier, but that was it. I had never taken care of anyone with an ostomy, nor (to my knowledge) known anyone with this unfamiliar rearrangement of internal plumbing. All I had was a vague memory of some organization for people with ostomies.

A couple of phone calls later, I discovered that the local chapter of the United Ostomy Association, which met in San Francisco once every two months, was meeting that night. And what a meeting! It was the breath of hope I sought: There *was* life after an ostomy! *Good, full life*. I was wrong: an ostomy wasn't the worst thing that could happen to someone.

When Mother entered the hospital, my life took on the pace — if not the laughs — of a Keystone Cops comedy. The doctors first scheduled Mother's surgery for Thursday—the day I had to be in Sacramento taking the *surgery* test for my nursing State Boards (the two days of licensing examinations that one must pass to become a registered nurse). For assorted reasons, including my pleas, the surgeons postponed the operation until 7:00 a.m. Monday. I still remember very little about the Boards (but I did pass).

Sunday evening, a telegram arrived from my brother-in-law and his family in Indonesia: "Arriving San Francisco International 8:00 a.m. Monday."

I promptly burst into tears. "Tell me this isn't happening," I howled to Art, my husband. Later, I would be able to laugh. But not yet.

After a dawn visit to the hospital, staying until Mother's pre-operative medication relaxed her, I scrambled out to the airport to meet my exhausted in-laws, including two babies. I fear I was less than the perfect hostess.

Bless Dick and Judy, weary as they were, for being so understanding during their visit. And bless my friend Marcia, who showed up at the hospital to share the vigil outside the operating room. And Art and our children who, while facing their own feelings about Grandma's illness, helped so much.

In some ways, the pace of those few days cushioned the event for me. I had so many other things to worry about that I didn't have to face what was happening to Mother or how I was reacting to it.

Sometimes I retreated into my brand new "nurse" self when it became too painful to be a "daughter" self. The "nurse" self tried to encourage Mother to talk about what she was feeling—when the "daughter" self didn't necessarily want to hear. And occasionally, I fear, the plain old "me" self got lost in the shuffle.

But I did the "right" things, said the "right" words — and congratulated myself on how beautifully I was coping. I really was handling this *very* well.

Hah!

As my friend Carol says, "What 'I'm really handling this well' means is 'I haven't even begun to face this problem yet'!"

How right she is. My comeuppance came quickly. Three days later, a woman died on our ward. It was the first time I had ever been with a dying person—and she happened to be exactly the same age as my mother, and to have the same diagnosis. Woodenly, I carried out the tasks afterward.

When my work shift ended, I walked out to the parking lot. The tears began streaming.

For a week, I couldn't walk into the hospital without starting to cry. I wore a rut between the front door and the nearest bathroom, where I would sit and bawl.

But eventually I was all cried out.

One day, the food tasted like corrugated cardboard and paste. The next day, it was real food again, the chicken succulent with herbs, the salad crisp and delicious. San Francisco isn't exactly noted for its tree-lined streets, but what trees and blooms there were—I was *seeing*.

It was as if by confronting my worst fears—unwillingly, to be sure—I had begun to move through them and beyond them. Only then could I start concentrating on *today*, with its many joys and victories.

I kept asking myself why *I* hurt so much. After all, it was Mother who was miserable those first days after surgery, Mother who was having to learn all about living with an ostomy (although the ostomy itself was surprisingly little bother), Mother who was living with a scary diagnosis.

But we relatives and spouses and friends hurt too and there doesn't seem to be any way to bypass that grieving. Instead, we struggle to find a path through it and beyond it. There are no "good" ways or "bad" ways—we are all different persons and our ways must be our own.

Why do we hurt? For many reasons.

Illness is itself a change and it brings about other changes. Relationships shift; that person we've always counted on—is now depending on us. We may feel left in the lurch, with crushing responsibilities and no one to share them. When someone close to us becomes seriously ill, we see our own vulnerability and mortality. That is frightening indeed. And we feel *with* the person who is ill, sharing the sorrow and the anger that this has happened.

If all that weren't enough, we may feel anger *at* this person for being ill—for disrupting our lives, for worrying us, for draining our time, perhaps, or our energy and resources.

That anger may be quite normal—but it's pretty hard to accept in ourselves. After all, how can we be angry at someone for being sick? Enter the guilt.

I wish I could say I have it all figured out. I don't. All those nice pigeonholed "stages" of grieving that my nursing textbooks warned me about—were never that neat.

They still aren't.

Feelings—my feelings anyway—tend to be a hodgepodge of sadness and fear, with generous dollops of anger, resentment, and sometimes self-pity thrown in. Not to mention guilt—for all that anger, resentment, and self-pity!

Sometimes I get exasperated and sometimes I get plain furious: "Why does she have to question *everything*?" or "Why did this have to happen?"

But time and tears have helped.

Now, often, there's a real sharing, of thoughts, of feelings, of those wispy flights of fancy, of terrible jokes—and of a deep love. That edge of illness makes the good times far sweeter.

I'm proud of my mother, for what she's done, how she's coped, what she *is*.

She may be missing a section of her intestine.

But she's got *plenty* of guts.

Addresses To Know

American Cancer Society
  777 Third Avenue
  New York, NY 10017
  (212) 371-2900   (local chapters in towns and cities)

Canadian Cancer Society
  25 Adelaide St. East
  Toronto 210 Ontario
  Canada
  (416) 364-7483   (local chapters in towns and cities)

Consumer Information Center
  Dept. 648 G
  Pueblo, Colorado 81009

International Association for Enterostomal Therapy
  505 N. Tustin Street, Suite 219
  Santa Ana, CA 92705
  (714) 541-5227

International Association for Medical Assistance to Travelers
(IAMAT)
  350 Fifth Avenue
  New York, NY 10001
  (212) 279-6465

International Ostomy Association
Check United Ostomy Association for current address

National Foundation for Ileitis & Colitis, Inc.
  295 Madison Avenue
  New York, NY 10017
  (212) 685-3440   (some local chapters)

Ileostomy Association
Central Office
Amblehurst House
Chobham, WOKING
Surrey GU24 8PZ

United Ostomy Association (Canadian Office)
409 Tache Avenue
Winnipeg, Manitoba
Canada R2H 2A6
(204) 237-2022

United Ostomy Association (U.S. Office)
2001 W. Beverly Boulevard
Los Angeles, CA 90057
(213) 413-5510   (local chapters in towns and cities)

GLOSSARY

ABDOMINO-PERINEAL RESECTION. (A-P Resection). Surgical procedure in which sigmoid colon and entire rectum and anus are removed. End of remaining colon is then brought out as permanent colostomy.

APPLIANCE. Pouch or device worn over stoma to collect feces or urine. Two basic types: disposable (single-use, temporary, expendable), worn for several days and then discarded; reusable, washed and stored between wearings.

BARIUM ENEMA. Special x-ray study of colon. Thick liquid substance inserted through anus or, in case of person with colostomy, through stoma, fills large intestine and makes it show up clearly on x-ray films taken during procedure. Barium enemas are *not* done for ileostomates.

BIOPSY. Examination of tissue removed from living body. Done to determine whether tumor is cancerous or not. Also done to discover other disease processes.

BLOCKAGE. Obstruction in digestive or urinary tract. Digestive tract blockage comes from undigested food or from tumor, trauma, or surgical damage. Urinary tract blockage is often a birth defect or may come from tumor or trauma.

COLECTOMY. Removal of part of colon.

COLITIS. Inflammation of colon (large intestine).

COLONIC CONDUIT. One kind of operation to divert urine away from bladder. Short section of colon is cut away, along with its blood and nerve supply. Section is closed at one end, ureters are attached to it, and open end is brought through abdominal wall to form stoma. Section thus becomes conduit, or passageway, for urine to outside body. Remaining ends of intestine are reconnected and resume function of moving feces out of body.

COLOSTOMY. Surgical opening of colon (large intestine).

Permanent colostomy. Usually involves loss of part of colon and, in most cases, rectum. Portion of remaining colon is brought through abdominal wall to form single stoma.

Temporary colostomy. Usually performed to allow lower part of colon and/or rectum to heal or rest. Two openings: right one discharges waste, left one only mucus. Stomas constructed in two ways:

Double-barrel colostomy. Two separate stomas may or may not be separated by skin. If segment of colon has been removed, stomas may be distant from each other.

Loop colostomy. Loop of intestine brought through hole in abdominal wall. Outside of loop is slit to create single stoma with openings to right and left. Right opening discharges waste, left only mucus.

Sigmoid colostomy. Surgical opening in upper end of sigmoid colon. Similar to descending colostomy but in descending colostomy opening is farther up, in descending colon. Most common colostomy. Stoma on left side of abdomen. May be permanent or temporary.

Transverse colostomy. Opening in transverse colon. Stoma located on upper abdomen, middle or to right. Usually temporary procedure, reconnected later. Occasionally permanent, following removal of all or most of colon beyond it.

CONTINENT ILEOSTOMY. Surgical variation on ileostomy. Surgeon loops part of ileum back on itself and constructs from loop a reservoir pouch inside abdomen. Doctor builds one-way valve from reservoir through abdominal wall; ostomate inserts catheter few times each day to drain feces from reservoir. To date, operation suitable only for a limited number of ileostomates.

CROHN'S DISEASE. (Ileitis, regional enteritis, or granulomatous disease of bowel). Inflammatory bowel disease, attacks deep lining of any part of small or large bowel. In selected cases, ileostomy becomes necessary.

DIAGNOSIS. Method of recognizing and identifying disease.

DIGESTIVE TRACT. (Alimentary canal). Consists of mouth, esophagus, stomach, small intestine, large intestine (colon), rectum, and anus.

Small intestine. Approximately 20 feet of coiled bowel consisting of *duodenum*, 10-12 inches long, beginning at outlet of stomach; *jejunum*, about 8 feet long; *ileum*, about 12 feet long, connecting to large intestine at pouch called *cecum*.

Large intestine (colon). Approximately six feet of large bowel beginning with cecum in right lower abdomen, ascending to right rib area *(ascending colon)*, crossing to left rib area *(transverse colon)*, descending along left side *(descending colon)*, slanting across left groin to mid-pelvis *(sigmoid colon)*, descending along spine *(rectum)* to outlet *(anus)*.

DIVERTICULITIS. Inflammation of pouches found in diverticulosis. May lead to temporary transverse colostomy.

DIVERTICULOSIS. Abnormal out-pouching of bowel wall, found frequently in people over 40. Usually gives no trouble.

ELECTROLYTES. Normal chemicals (such as salt) dissolved in body fluids. Needed in small amounts to maintain body activity. If electrolytes are out of balance, person may become ill and weak, may need to take chemicals by mouth or through vein.

ENCRUSTATION. "Warty" looking, gray raised area sometimes appearing on skin around urinary stomas; caused by alkaline urine bathing skin.

ENTERITIS. Any inflammation of intestine.

ENTEROSTOMAL THERAPIST. Nurse or technician who has received formal training in management of all types of stomas and draining wounds and whose competency has been certified by International Association for Enterostomal Therapy.

EXCORIATION. For ostomates, refers to red, raw-appearing, sore skin around stoma, usually caused by enzymes in feces or by urine eroding skin surface, or by abuse of skin by scrubbing or scratching.

EXSTROPHY OF BLADDER. Birth defect. Bladder on outside of body, "turned inside out" so urine drips continuously from exposed organ. Sometimes treated with urinary diversion.

FAMILIAL POLYPOSIS (multiple polyps). Rare disease, runs in families, in which colon and rectum contain large numbers of polyps.

Tend to become cancerous if colon and rectum are not removed during early adulthood.

FECES. Bodily wastes which are discharged through anus or colostomy and ileostomy stomas.

FIBEROPTIC COLONOSCOPY. Visual examination of part or all of colon with fiberoptic colonoscope, lighted flexible tube several feet in length which can be passed around loops and curves of colon. Polyps can be removed through instrument.

HERNIA. Bulging to loop or knuckle of body organ or tissue through structure which usually contains it. For ostomates, protrusion of intestine through muscle of abdomen, sometimes around stoma.

ILEAL CONDUIT (Bricker Loop, Ileal Loop). Operation which allows urine to pass from kidneys through passageway made of short segment of small intestine (ileum) to outside of body. Performed when patient's bladder may no longer be used because of disease or defect. Similar to colonic conduit except that section of small intestine is used for conduit.

ILEITIS. Inflammation of the small intestine (ileum).

ILEOSTOMY. Surgical opening in ileum portion of small intestine. Entire colon and rectum may be removed; rectum sometimes remains. End portion of ileum is brought through abdominal wall to form stoma, usually on lower right side of abdomen. Feces eliminated through stoma. Except in continent ileostomy, appliance must be worn at all times to collect feces. Where part of colon remains, there may be a second stoma to left of ileostomy stoma; this stoma secretes only mucus.

IMPOTENCE. In male only, inability to achieve or sustain erection.

INCONTINENCE. Inability to control elimination of urine or feces.

INFLAMMATORY BOWEL DISEASE. Catch-all term for several diseases which attack intestinal tract. Most common diseases are ulcerative colitis, Crohn's disease.

IRRIGATION. For colostomates, an enema through the stoma. Water distends bowel, causes bowel to expel wastes.

IVP (Intravenous pyelogram). X-ray of kidneys and urinary passages to show any blockage or abnormality. Medicine is injected into the vein so kidneys, ureters, and bladder, which normally do not show in x-ray, can be seen.

KARAYA. Water-soluble, gummy substance used for healing or preventing damage to skin. Comes in gelatinous sheets, powder, paste; used as skin barrier around stoma.

KOCK POUCH. One kind of continent ileostomy, named after Nils Kock, Swedish surgeon who devised procedure.

MAGNETIC PLUG. Experimental variation on sigmoid colostomy. Magnetic ring, wrapped in plastic, implanted in fatty area around flush stoma, holds metal magnetic disc firmly over colostomy so feces and gas cannot escape. To discharge feces, person removes outer cap, allows feces to pass, and replaces cap. No appliance necessary.

OSTOMY. Surgical opening. Shortened form of description for colostomy, ileostomy, urostomy.

PERINEAL WOUND. (Posterior wound). Large gap where anus used to be. Occurs when rectum and anus are removed in ileostomy and colostomy surgery. Heals slowly as new tissue fills area.

PERISTALSIS. Progressive movement of intestine by which contents are pushed toward outlet.

pH OF URINE. How acid or alkaline urine is.

POLYP. Small projection inside bowel. Occasionally cancerous.

PROGNOSIS. Probable outcome of disease or other event.

PROLAPSE. "Falling out" or protrusion of stoma end of intestine from the body.

RETRACTION. Condition in which stoma draws back into body.

SIGMOIDOSCOPY. Visual examination with 10-inch or longer lighted tube of anus, rectum, lower part of sigmoid colon.

SKIN BARRIER. Any one of several substances used to cover skin around stoma to protect it from feces or urine. Can be pliable sheets, powders, pastes, sprays, etc.

SPHINCTER. Ringlike muscle surrounding a passageway of organ and able to open and close. Sphincter in anus provides bowel control; bladder sphincter controls urine.

STOMA. End of ureter, ileum or colon which can be seen coming through the skin. Often protrudes ½'' to 1¼'' or longer.

ULCERATIVE COLITIS. Inflammation of the colon (large intestine), in which ulcers form in intestinal lining. Severe diarrhea is primary symptom of disease, which occurs most often in young adults. Severe cases may lead to ileostomy.

UNDIVERSION. Reconnection of the urinary tract after a urinary diversion in which bladder remains, to eliminate stoma and permit passage of urine through normal opening.

URINARY TRACT. System in body composed of *kidney, ureters* (tubes connecting kidneys to bladder), *bladder,* and *urethra* (tube leading from bladder to outside of body. Urine is made in kidneys, passes down ureters, is collected in bladder, and passes outside through urethra.

UROSTOMY. (Urinary diversion). Any one of several surgical procedures to divert urine away from diseased or defective ureters, bladder or urethra. In urostomy, new passageway for urine is formed through abdominal wall to outside body. Appliances are worn with all urostomies. Urostomies include:
Nephrostomy. Tube inserted from outside abdominal wall into kidney to drain urine. Almost always temporary ostomy.
Ureterostomy. One or both ureters are brought through abdominal wall. Temporary or permanent ostomy.
Ileal or *Colonic conduit* (defined earlier).
Vesicostomy. Bladder is brought to abdominal wall and opening constructed directly from bladder to outside the body.